THE
ELI'S CHEESECAKE
COOKBOOK

THE
ELI'S CHEESECAKE
COOKBOOK

REMARKABLE RECIPES *from a* CHICAGO LEGEND

MAUREEN SCHULMAN · TARA LANE

DIANA MOLES · JOLENE WORTHINGTON

Food photography by Peter McCullough.

Printed in China.

Library of Congress Cataloging-in-Publication Data

Schulman, Maureen.
 The Eli's Cheesecake cookbook : remarkable recipes from a Chicago legend / Maureen
Schulman, Tara Lane, Jolene Worthington, Diana Moles.
     pages cm
 Includes index.
 Summary: "A cookbook celebrating the 35th anniversary of the Chicago restaurant Eli's
Cheesecake, including recipes, anecdotes, and photographs"-- Provided by publisher.
 ISBN 978-1-57284-182-6 (hard cover) -- ISBN 1-57284-182-6 (hard cover) -- ISBN
978-1-57284-769-9 (ebook) -- ISBN 1-57284-769-7 (ebook)
 1. Cheesecake. 2. Eli's Cheesecake World. I. Lane, Tara. II. Worthington, Jolene. III.
Moles, Diana. IV. Title.
 TX773.S3335 2015
 641.86'53--dc23

                              2015031420

10 9 8 7 6 5 4 3 2 1

Midway is an imprint of Agate Publishing. Agate books are available in bulk at discount
prices. For more information, go to agatepublishing.com.

DEDICATED WITH LOVE TO ELI SCHULMAN, a larger-than-life, one-in-a-million guy with a twinkle in his eye who captured the heart of Chicago with his amazing food and effervescent personality. Eli would be so happy that his cheesecake legacy remains strong, and that no one will ever say "Eli who?" Everyone at The Eli's Cheesecake Company, a family-owned business, continues to be inspired by Eli's magic and strives for excellence every day.

This year marks Eli's Cheesecake's 35th anniversary, which was the driving force behind the creation of this book. We are so happy that you have decided to cook with us!

This is your chance to peek inside the legendary kitchens of Eli's The Place For Steak and the Eli's Cheesecake bakery, and learn how to make the most popular recipes from these icons of the Chicago food scene. Our goal is to provide you with the scientific knowledge and detailed recipes necessary to bake a perfect cheesecake, all while learning about Eli Schulman's storied rise to top restaurateur and baker extraordinaire. Whether you're a cook, baker, or Chicago history buff or simply have fond memories of dining at one of Eli's restaurants, this book is filled with historical photos, celebrity snapshots, and lots of big cakes, as well as clear and beautiful step-by-step food photography for every recipe.

GOOD THINGS TO EAT
ELI'S
ogden huddle
ARGYLE ST., & SHERIDAN RD.
CHICAGO
CLOSE COVER BEFORE STRIKING

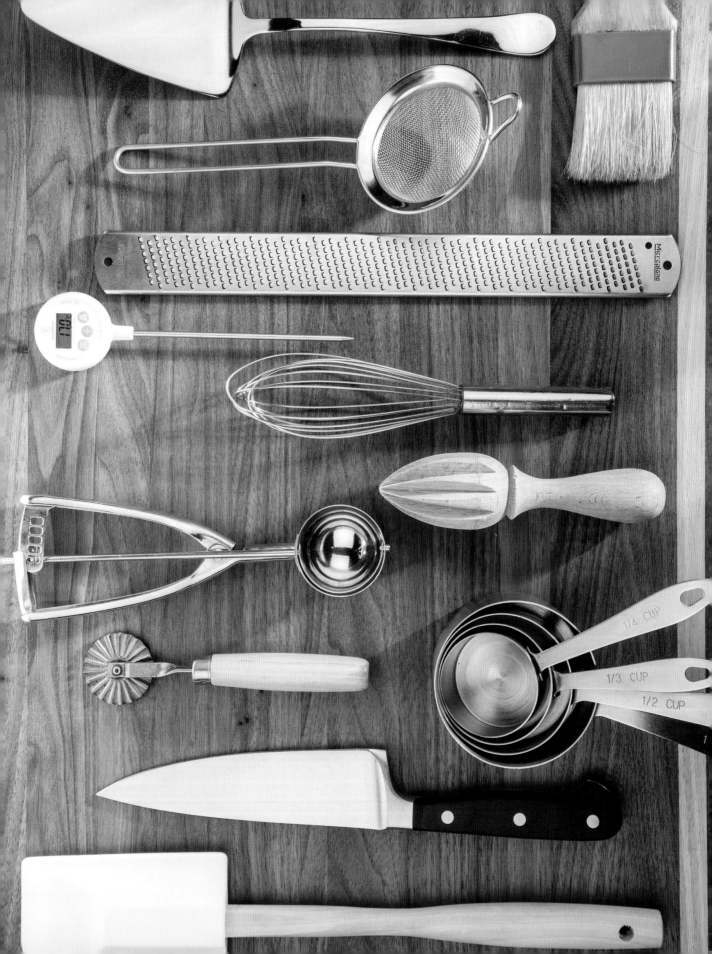

CONTENTS

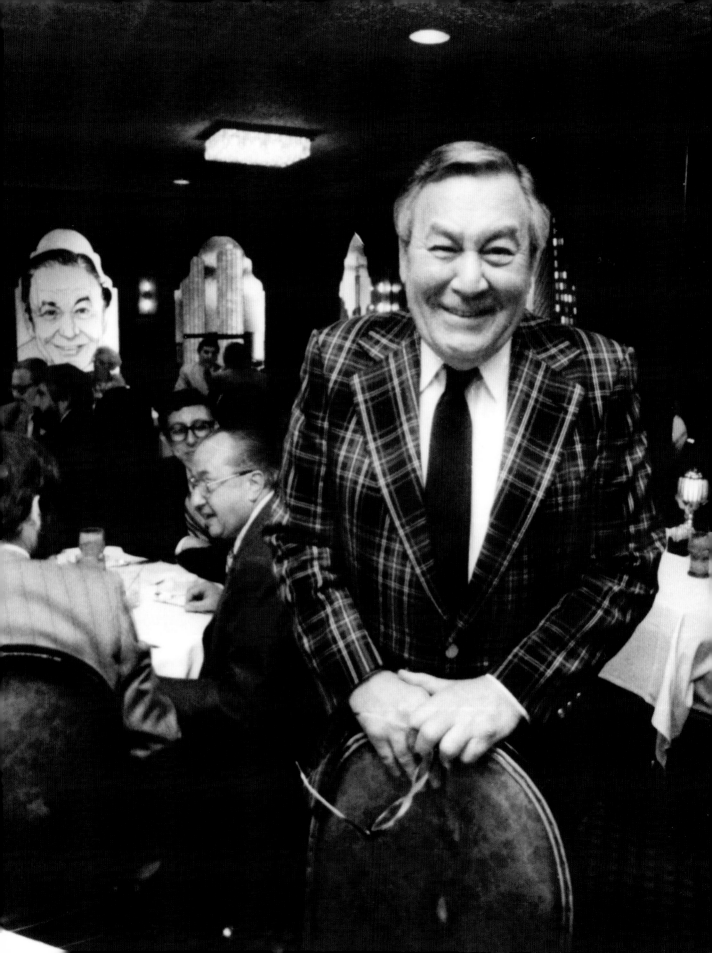

FOREWORD

I LIKE TO THINK OF ELI AS HE WAS IN LIFE. Though he died in 1988, I still like to think of Eli as alive. The man was so full of life that it's not a great leap to imagine him still with us today. I like to imagine the smile that would cross his face as he surveyed the accomplishments of his three granddaughters, all grown and beautiful.

Would Eli smile? Sure, he would. He smiled a lot. He smiled the last time we sat together, at Eli's The Place For Steak. It was a couple of months before he died, and he was in a reflective mood. He told me, "It's been the best…and the worst. I've met so many people, made so many friends. But as you get older, you start to see them drop off, like leaves from a tree. But to have come from where I came from, to have known the people I've known…I'd have to say that I'm the luckiest man in the world."

Eli smiles with delight in the dining room.

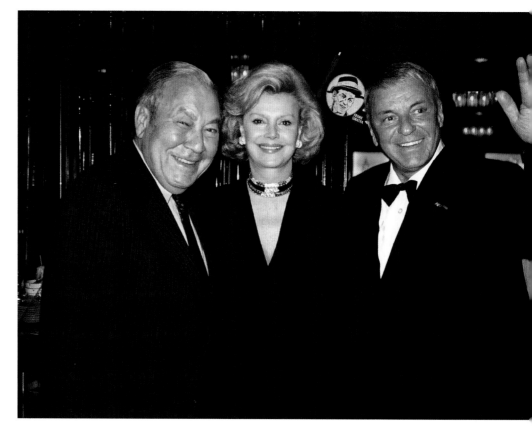

Eli with Barbara and Frank Sinatra at Eli's. During that visit, Frank invited all of us to his show. Eli decided not to go because he wanted to make sure everything was perfect at the restaurant for the arrival of Frank and his entourage. Frank spied Eli's empty seat in the audience and sent his wife out to find out where Eli was. Marc and Maureen told her that he was in the bathroom and quickly called him from a pay phone (this was in the days before cell phones) to tell him to race over—and he did.

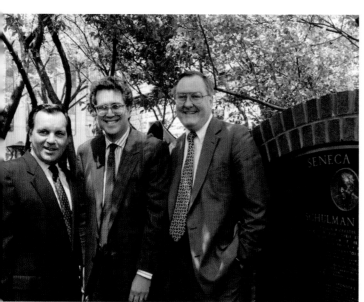

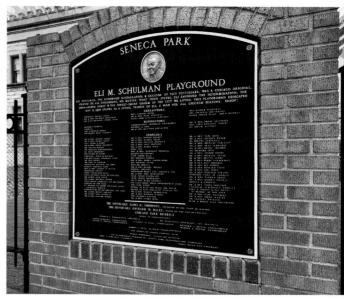

FROM LEFT: *Opening of the Eli M. Schulman Playground with Mayor Richard M. Daley, Marc Schulman, and Illinois Governor James R Thompson; Eli's plaque in the Seneca Park Eli Schulman Playground.*

"Leaves from a tree," he said again, and immediately I realized that the trees closest to where Eli spent most of his time—in his restaurant—were just across Chicago Avenue, a few steps away, dotting Seneca Park and its small playground. That small patch of green for decades provided a peaceful place, an especially quiet slice of the city, sitting amid the bustle of shoppers and strollers in the shadows of high-rises. There, Eli would often sit and watch little children at play. Sometimes he would talk to them, and his kindly face would come alive. His eyes would sparkle. The little kids at the park, if they thought about him at all, probably considered him to be just some nice old guy. He was all that, and more. Former Bears' coach Mike Ditka once said of him, "To know this man was to love him." Eli could talk with anyone. He listened. He cared. And he was an enthralling storyteller. Even in the center of his star-studded milieu, he exemplified simple values: friendship and honesty, Chicago style. Few knew that the watch he wore was a gift from Frank Sinatra.

Eli was a poor kid from the Greater Lawndale area on the city's West Side. There was not much time for playing in parks for him; his dad died when he was young, and from then on, Eli had to work hard. He sold 10-cent windup toys on street corners and seat cushions at the City's baseball yards, hawked newspapers, and delivered packages. He made it, and he made it big. His restaurants were patronized by famous and influential people. Some of them were good people, and most were his friends, too.

I regret not spending more time with Eli in the park by his restaurant, and never having the chance to go to the track with him—the ponies were his special passion. But I was at the restaurant often enough to observe him in his element. There, he was something to behold, moving from table to table, chatting, joking, making new friends. It was, of course, a gathering place for luminaries from the worlds of sports, show business, and politics—especially politics. They were drawn as much by the food as by the owner's magnetic personality.

In the pages that follow, Eli's daughter-in-law Maureen, wife of his only son, Marc, will share a much more detailed biography of this great man. What you'll read there would make Eli smile, too. He'd be so happy to know how well Marc and Maureen have lived their lives, and how they and others have turned his modest little idea for a new dessert into an international sensation. Today, Eli's cheesecake is a favorite after-dinner treat for current and former presidents, and perhaps future ones as well, since Hillary Clinton enjoyed some at her 50th birthday party. I like Eli's cheesecake, too, and am continually surprised by its variations. I can get it almost anywhere, any time these days.

I can just imagine the smile Eli would have had on the cold February morning when a group gathered under a large tent in the park by his restaurant. They were there to celebrate the news that the park's playground would be renamed in Eli's memory, and to announce that money would be raised to rebuild the playground and to reconstruct the entire park. Eli's The Place For Steak is gone now, replaced by the Lurie Children's Hospital. It's a fitting transformation, and something else that would make Eli smile. In that playground across the street, which now bears his name, he'd find a plaque bearing his likeness and these words: "Eli Schulman, the renowned restaurateur and creator of Eli's Cheesecake, was a Chicago original. Friend to all Chicagoans, no matter what their status, Eli embodies the determination, the open-armed spirit and the street-smart charm of the City he loved. This playground, dedicated May 7, 1990, stands as a living tribute to Eli, a man for all Chicago seasons. Enjoy!"

I love that still today, Eli could wander over and find his park filled with kids and their laughter and smiles. Life goes on. **—RICK KOGAN**

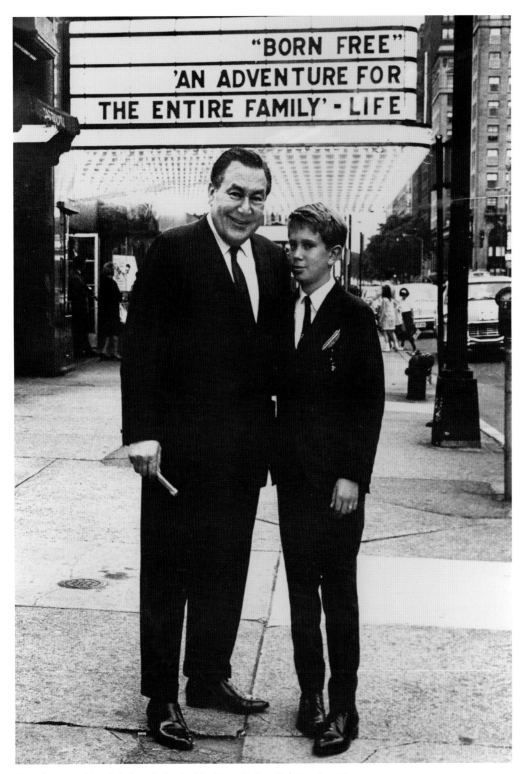

Eli and a young Marc Schulman in front of the Stage Deli on Oak Street, 1966.

Eli's Ogden Huddle, Eli's first restaurant, 1940.

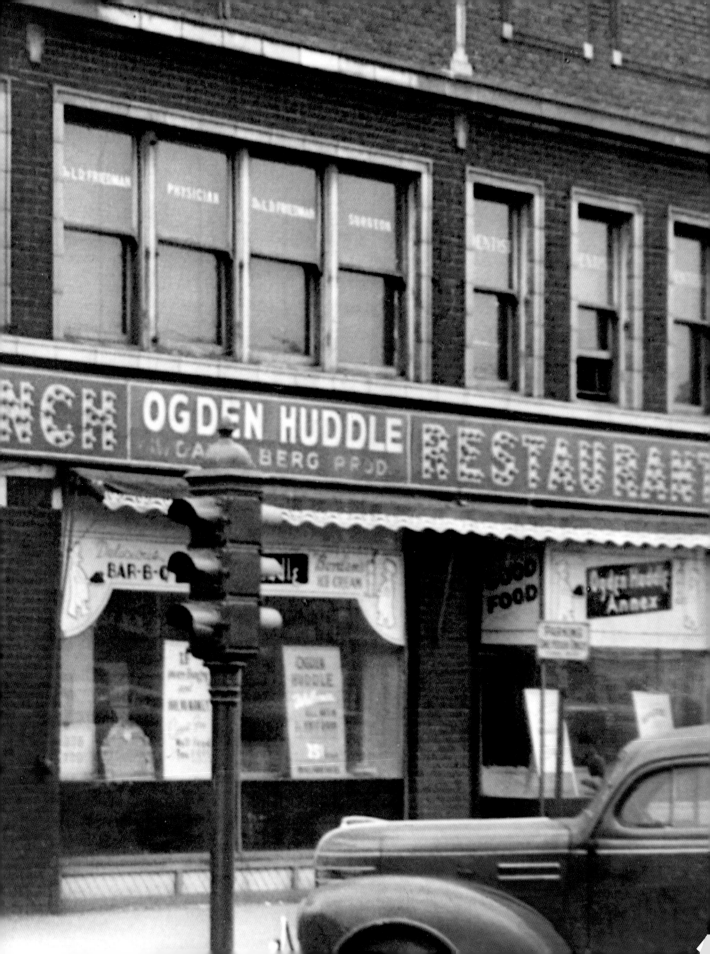

ELI'S STORY

IN 1978, ELI SCHULMAN DECIDED TO MAKE CHEESECAKE THE signature dessert at his famous Chicago restaurant, Eli's The Place For Steak. He also decided to make it himself—his own recipe, unlike any others he had tasted. So how did a man with no formal culinary or pastry training wind up creating one of the country's best loved cheesecakes for one of the most popular restaurants in Chicago?

Well, first of all, we're talking about Eli Schulman, a diamond-in-the-rough kind of guy who needed no last name to be identified. Everyone from movie stars and politicians to the guy selling newspapers on the corner simply called him Eli. A celebrity in his own right, Eli was on the inside track of everything. He was everyone's best friend and confidante, and Chicago's go-to guy.

Eli showing off two beautiful slices of cheesecake at Eli's The Place For Steak, where he invented the dessert.

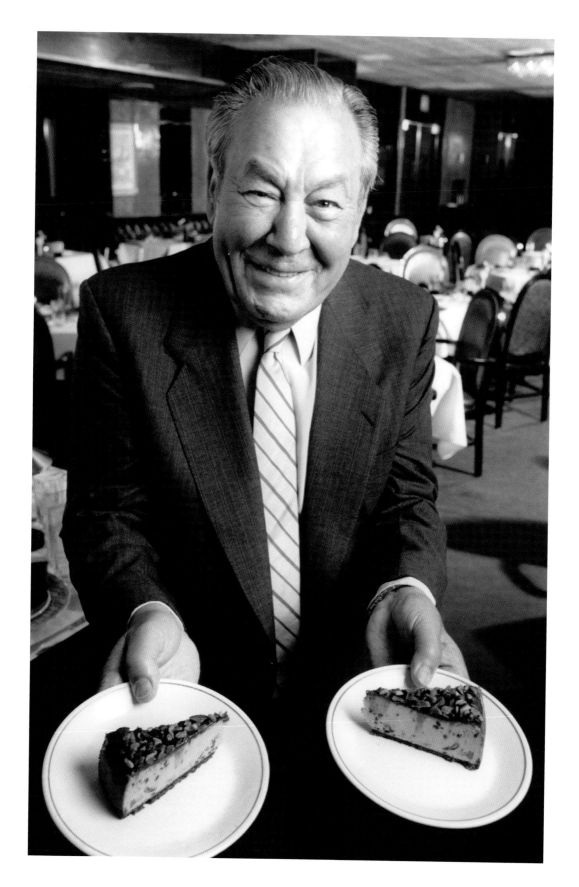

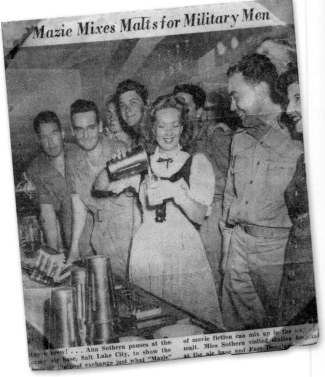

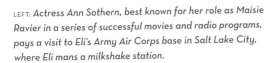

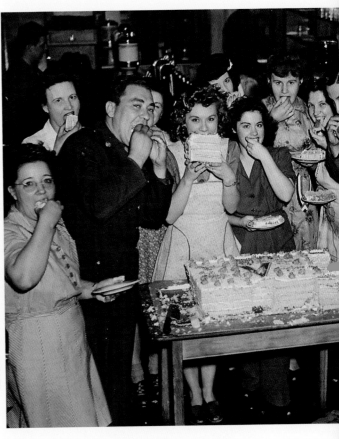

LEFT: *Actress Ann Sothern, best known for her role as Maisie Ravier in a series of successful movies and radio programs, pays a visit to Eli's Army Air Corps base in Salt Lake City, where Eli mans a milkshake station.*

RIGHT: *Eli with a Big Cake at his Army Air Corps base in Salt Lake City, Utah, during World War II. There, Eli honed his baking skills, and this pretty cake is a good example of his work.*

Eli's irresistible charm made people clamor for his attention. The ultimate honor: Eli would sit down at a table, rip the menu in half, and announce, "You've made decisions all day...I'll order for you."

When Eli was only 16, his father, a baker, died suddenly. Eli was forced to drop out of school and find work in order to help support his mother, brother, and three sisters. Like many other hardworking people living on Chicago's West Side, Eli held every job under the sun to make ends meet—selling shoes out of the back of a car, working a booth at the Maxwell Street Market, and eventually serving as a 29th Ward precinct captain.

Eli's debut in the restaurant business was a bit unconventional. The year was 1940, and he spied a foreclosure notice on the door of a coffee shop he frequented at Ogden and Kedzie. Inspired, he bought the building and restaurant on the spot and renamed it Eli's Ogden Huddle.

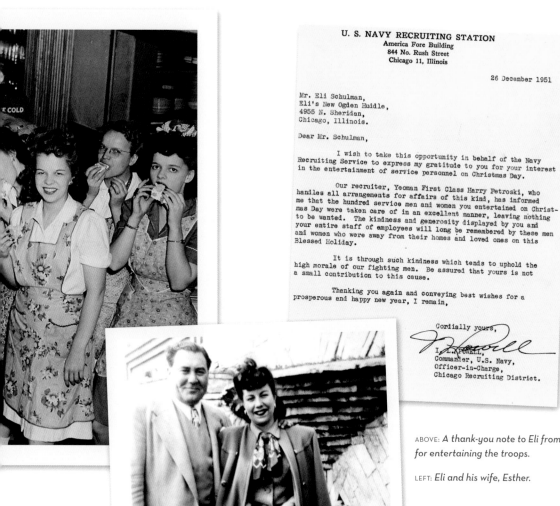

U. S. NAVY RECRUITING STATION
America Fore Building
844 No. Rush Street
Chicago 11, Illinois

26 December 1951

Mr. Eli Schulman,
Eli's New Ogden Huddle,
4955 N. Sheridan,
Chicago, Illinois.

Dear Mr. Schulman,

I wish to take this opportunity in behalf of the Navy Recruiting Service to express my gratitude to you for your interest in the entertainment of service personnel on Christmas Day.

Our recruiter, Yeoman First Class Harry Petroski, who handles all arrangements for affairs of this kind, has informed me that the hundred service men and women you entertained on Christmas Day were taken care of in an excellent manner, leaving nothing to be wanted. The kindness and generosity displayed by you and your entire staff of employees will long be remembered by these men and women who were away from their homes and loved ones on this Blessed Holiday.

It is through such kindness which tends to uphold the high morale of our fighting men. Be assured that yours is not a small contribution to this cause.

Thanking you again and conveying best wishes for a prosperous and happy new year, I remain,

Cordially yours,

I. L. POWELL,
Commander, U.S. Navy,
Officer-in-Charge,
Chicago Recruiting District.

ABOVE: *A thank-you note to Eli from the US Navy for entertaining the troops.*

LEFT: *Eli and his wife, Esther.*

On the restaurant's scheduled opening day, Eli arrived and found the cook passed out drunk on the floor. Customers were arriving, so Eli had no choice but to open. The first order was a breaded veal cutlet. Eli had no idea how to make one, so he hurried back to the kitchen and called his mother to get the recipe. He made his mother's veal cutlet, the customer loved it, and the rest is history. Soon after, Eli hired a new cook. Eventually, his first customer returned and ordered the same dish—and told him that he liked the veal cutlet he had the first day even better. Eli had a feel for food. If he could dream it, he could make it.

At one point, Eli hung a sign in the restaurant's window: "If you are hungry and have no money, come in. We will feed you." He meant to keep it there for only a short time, but it ended up staying there for a dozen years. Eli said that in all that time, he never encountered a single faker.

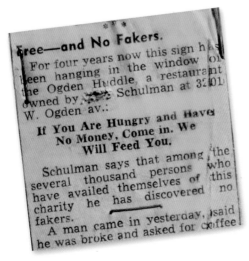

Generosity was Eli's signature characteristic. He set the tone that continues today at The Eli's Cheesecake Company. The company is firmly entrenched in the community, supporting hundreds of Chicago's not-for-profits.

A year later, Eli was drafted into the Army Air Corps. The Army turned out to be his culinary school of sorts. While Eli's brother Nate and sister Bertha ran Eli's Ogden Huddle, Eli ran air base restaurants in Texas, Colorado, and Utah. There, he learned to serve large numbers of people, baked cakes, and even finagled a way to run soft drinks through the water fountains.

After Eli returned from the Army, he married Esther Nettis, who worked with Eli throughout his career in the restaurant business. Nate and Bertha continued to run the West Side Huddle. Eli joined the mass exodus to the North Side and opened a second location at Argyle and Sheridan. After World War II, Chicago's North Side was booming: people were buying houses, having babies, and eating out. Eli's big personality and charitable heart quickly gained notoriety. At the same time, he maintained an interest in politics, serving as both a deputy coroner while running the restaurant and years later as a Commissioner of the North Shore Mosquito Abatement District.

In 1962, a few restaurants and odd jobs later, Eli made the big move to the Gold Coast. In that day, it was a mecca for showgirls, up-and-coming entertainers, young professionals, and scores of singles looking for a place to hang out. They found just the place: Eli's Stage Delicatessen at 50 E. Oak Street. The Deli served breakfast all day and all night, and its six-inch-high hand-cut hot corned beef sandwiches and Eli's great personality were a powerful draw. Quickly, Eli's had countless regulars, including local pols, columnists, the City's movers and shakers, and everyone from Woody Allen and Joan Rivers to Barbra

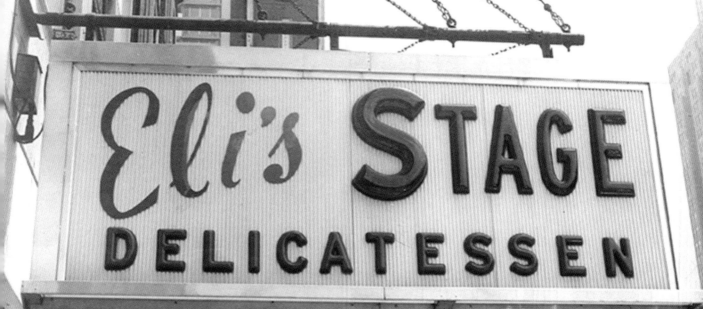

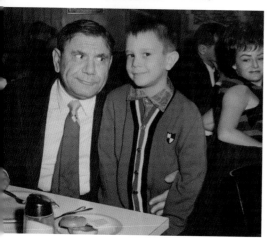

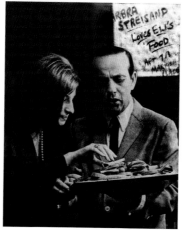

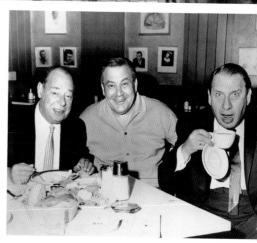

CLOCKWISE FROM THE TOP: *Eli's Stage Deli; in the background, the Esquire Theater sign features actress Eve Arden.*

Eli, comedian and singer Joe E. Lewis, and funnyman Henny Youngman pose at the Deli.

Barbra Streisand eats a corned beef sandwich at Eli's Stage Delicatessen. She was in town for some shows at Mr. Kelly's, a nightclub just down the street from the Deli.

Actor "Ooh! Ooh!" Joe E. Ross (Patrolman Gunther Toody on Car 54 Where Are You?) poses with Marc, age 7.

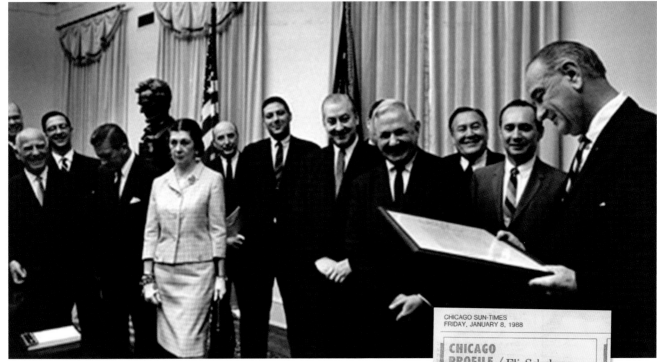

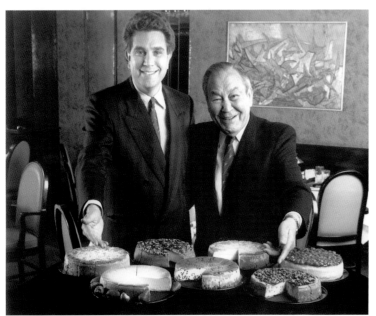

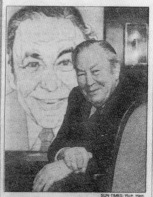

FROM TOP: *Eli with "Friends from Illinois: Land of Lincoln," presenting a bust of Abraham Lincoln to President Lyndon Johnson at the White House in 1967; Eli and Marc, a father-and-son team like no other, displaying Eli's Cheesecake at the restaurant.*

CHICAGO SUN-TIMES
FRIDAY, JANUARY 8, 1988

CHICAGO PROFILE / Eli Schulman

SUN-TIMES/Rich Hein

FAME CLAIM
He taught Chicago diners to love liver and cheesecake. He's among the last of the big-time personal Chicago restaurateurs.

JOB
He owns Eli's The Place for Steak, 215 E. Chicago, works there 10 to 14 hours daily, tries to stop at each table. Celebrity fans have included Frank Sinatra, Dinah Shore, Roger Moore, Leon Uris, Ingrid Bergman, Kup.

WHY LIVER AND CHEESECAKE?
"Remember how your mother made good things? I was at a club in Florida and ordered liver. The way it was described on the menu, it reminded me of my mother's. When the liver arrived, I didn't like it." He decided to re-create "dishes that came from old recipes, the kind our mothers made." After experimenting, he came up with his liver recipe. When he desired a good dessert, more experiments produced his cheesecake.

PHILOSOPHY
"Love is the name of the game. I love people. Without people I would be nobody. And my mother taught me, 'Charity will never bust you.'"

STATS
Grew up in Lawndale, dropped out of Marshall High. After his father died, he sold Christmas toys "at 10 below on street corners" at age 15. He became a Democratic precinct captain at 20 and remained one for many years. Lives Near North with Esther, his wife of 40 years. Son, Marc, founded Eli's, Chicago's Finest Cheesecake Inc. Its cheesecakes, based on Eli's recipe, are sold in 22 states.

Streisand and Bobby Short. At the Deli, Eli himself became a celebrity and a powerhouse. If it was happening in Chicago, Eli knew all about it.

The Deli was very successful, but Eli had yet another dream: a steakhouse. In 1966, while still running Eli's Stage Delicatessen, he opened Eli's The Place For Steak in the Carriage House Hotel, located at 215 E. Chicago Avenue. The Deli's regulars followed Eli to his new white-tablecloth restaurant, where they'd find a mound of chopped liver, vegetable crudités on ice, and a bread basket full of raisin pumpernickel and matzoh on each table. At Eli's The Place For Steak, liver haters became liver lovers thanks to the famous Liver Eli. And then there were those thick, juicy steaks; Shrimp a la Marc; Shrimp de Jonghe; and countless other dishes Eli imagined and made real.

Eli served various desserts through the years, including the ice cream snowball with coconut and chocolate sauce, apple strudel, and his least favorite dessert of all—fresh fruit. (He would say "It can look great, but taste like a potato... and that's the last thing people remember.") In the late '70s, he decided that cheesecake would be the signature dessert for Eli's The Place For Steak. Every day between the lunch and dinner service, he would head to the restaurant's kitchen to experiment with cheesecake recipes, and he'd often serve up test versions to regular customers to get their opinions.

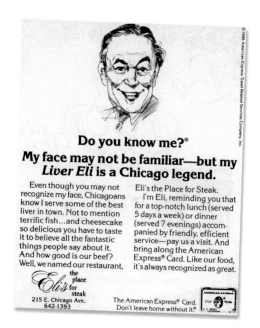

An American Express ad features the restaurant's famous Liver Eli.

After about a year of testing, Eli finalized four cheesecake recipes: original plain, chocolate chip, cinnamon raisin, and Hawaiian. At the time, Eli had no idea that he was about to change the world of cheesecake forever. Eli's cheesecake, a richer, creamier alternative to its New York counterpart, featured an all-butter-cookie crust instead of a graham cracker one. It was so deliciously different from other cheesecakes that Eli's is credited with creating a new class of cheesecake…Chicago Style.

The restaurant's customers loved the new dessert, but Eli wanted to test it in bigger waters. In 1980, he decided to offer the cheesecake at a booth at the first Taste of Chicago, a food festival dreamed up by his good friend and fellow restaurateur Arnie Morton and Chicago Mayor Jane Byrne. The first Taste was a single-day event, held on July 4 on Michigan Avenue in front of the Tribune Tower. No one knew what to expect. The street was packed with people, and Eli's booth was among the busiest. Eli feverishly cut cheesecake all day long, as fast as he could, all while wearing a suit and tie.

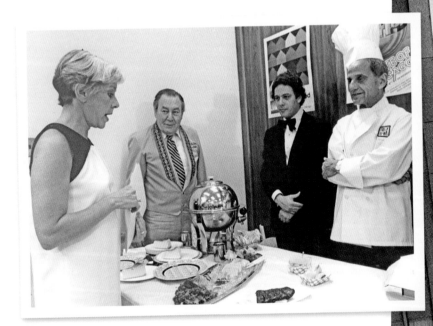

ABOVE: *Eli, Rich Melman, and Don Roth show Mayor Jane Byrne what they'll be selling at the first Taste of Chicago, July 4, 1980.*

RIGHT: *The first Taste of Chicago was a rousing success, if crowd size is any indication. Hundreds of thousands of people jammed a six-block stretch of Michigan Avenue, sampling foods from 40 restaurants—and, of course, Eli's cheesecake.*

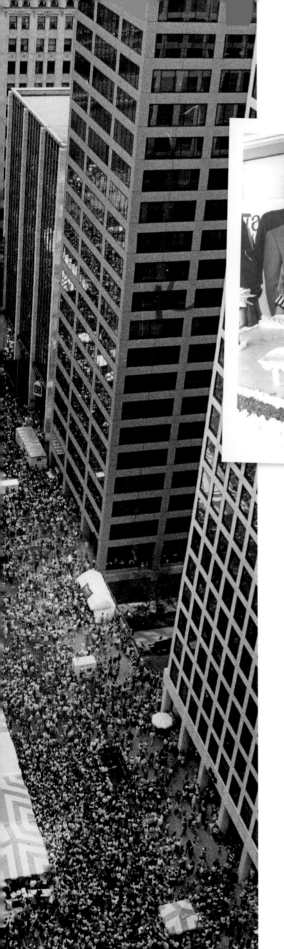

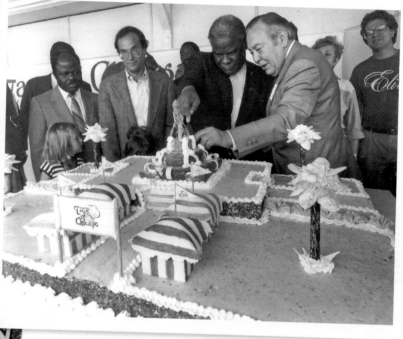

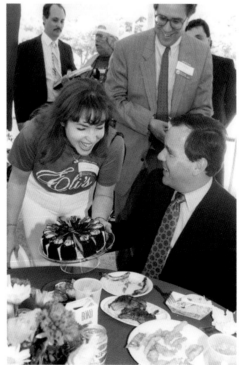

ABOVE: *Eli and Chicago Mayor Harold Washington at Taste of Chicago 1985 with a giant cheesecake replica of Chicago's Grant Park, complete with a buttercream-and-fondant Buckingham Fountain. Mayor Washington was a big Eli's Cheesecake fan; he even served it at his celebration in New Orleans when the Chicago Bears won the Super Bowl in 1986.*

LEFT: *Mayor Daley's first Taste of Chicago press party, in 1989. Maureen noticed he was eating lunch but had no dessert on the table...so she gathered up the nerve to bring him a whole turtle cheesecake.*

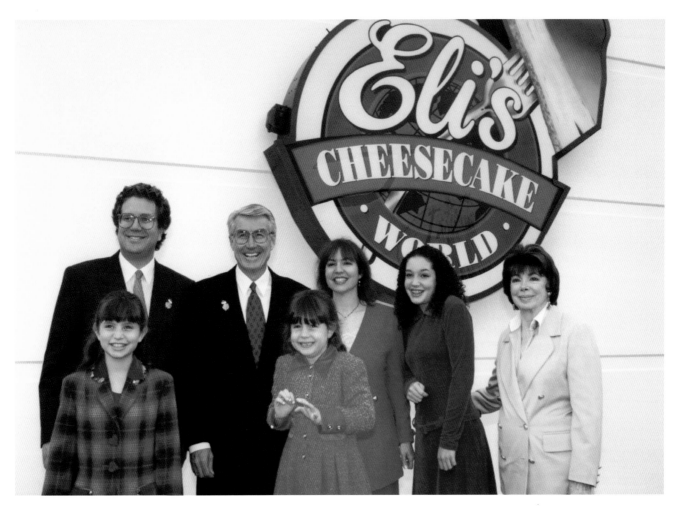

In October 1996, Eli's Cheesecake World, a state-of-the-art 62,000 sq. ft. bakery, retail store, and café, made its debut. Under the sign stands Eli's granddaughters Kori, Elana, and Haley, along with (left to right) Marc, Illinois Governor Jim Edgar, Maureen, and Maureen's mother, Harriet.

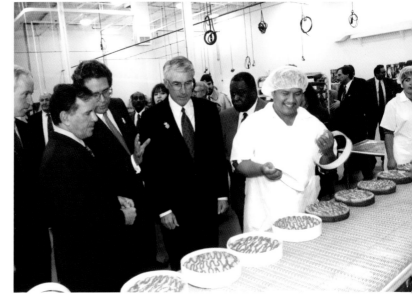

Marc gives an opening-day tour of Eli's Cheesecake World to Mayor Richard Daley and Illinois Governor Jim Edgar.

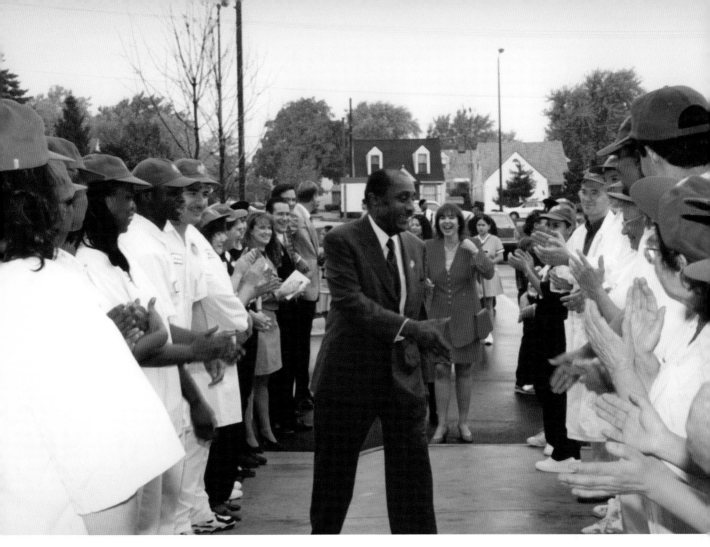

John H. Johnson, publisher and founder of the Johnson Publishing Company and Ebony and Jet magazines, at the opening of Eli's Cheesecake World.

After the Taste, many other restaurateurs wanted to serve Eli's cheesecake, but he couldn't produce enough cakes at the restaurant to keep up with demand. He was at a crossroads—make the cheesecakes for his restaurant and his restaurant alone, or begin a separate cheesecake business. Four years later, Eli's son, Marc Schulman (the namesake of Shrimp à la Marc), left behind a successful legal career to head up The Eli's Cheesecake Company. Initially, the company rented a bakery on Chicago's Northwest Side, but it grew quickly. In 1996, Eli's Cheesecake World, a 62,000 sq. ft. bakery, café, and retail store, opened at 6701 W. Forest Preserve Drive in Chicago.

From the very beginning, Marc knew that in order to be successful, he had to build the best pastry team possible. One of the first hires was Jolene Worthington, a talented pastry

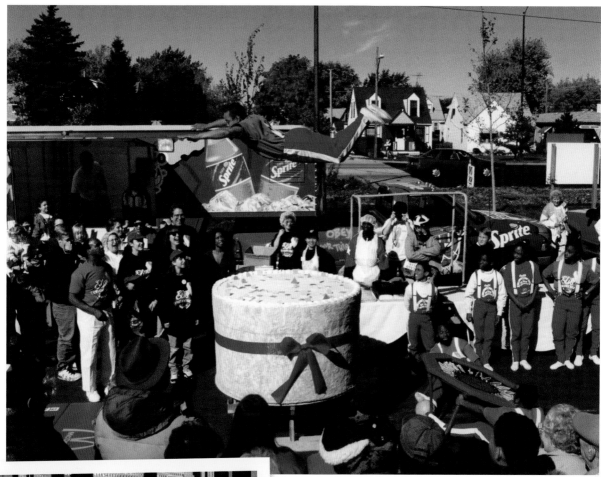

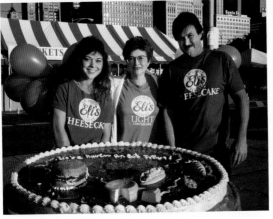

chef, author, and food writer (and a coauthor of this book). Jolene took a very good thing—Eli's original Chicago-style cheesecake recipe—and experimented until she had created nearly 50 varieties. She viewed cheesecake in a new way, as the most versatile dessert on the planet. She created many different interpretations, but all maintained Eli's signature taste and texture.

Marc believed that empowering Eli's associates was critical to the success of The Eli's Cheesecake Company. In the early 1990s, Eli's partnered with Wright College to implement

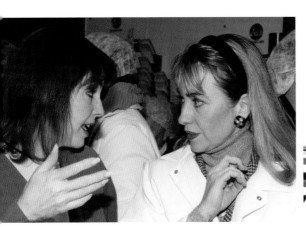

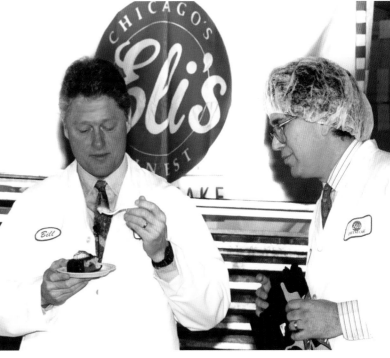

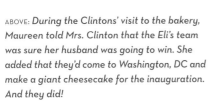

ABOVE: *During the Clintons' visit to the bakery, Maureen told Mrs. Clinton that the Eli's team was sure her husband was going to win. She added that they'd come to Washington, DC and make a giant cheesecake for the inauguration. And they did!*

a General Education Development (GED) program at the bakery. Eli's GED candidates took on-site classes three days per week while their coworkers covered for them. This allowed working parents the opportunity to gain a degree and still return home at a decent hour to be there for their families. The day before the 1992 Illinois primary, then-Arkansas Gov. Bill Clinton and Hillary Clinton came to Chicago and made a campaign stop at Eli's Cheesecake, precisely because of Eli's innovative education program. Clinton won Illinois, and we'd like to think the cheesecake helped!

In short, Jolene shepherded Eli's Chicago's Finest Cheesecake into the 21st century with finesse, seeking out the most specific and best ingredients and expanding her pastry and production team to include 25-year veterans Diana Moles (a coauthor of this cookbook) and Mike Newhouse. Jolene and Diana became cheesecake scientists, experimenting with Eli's baking practices and thinking outside the 9-inch round. They've made cheesecake in every form, from bite-sized squares to frozen on a stick to 2,000-pound rounds for four presidential inaugurations. Eli's Cheesecake uses cream cheese, of course, which Jolene refers to as "magical," but she also uses alternatives like goat cheese, quark, crème fraîche, and ricotta to surprise the taste buds. She and her team have been instrumental in turning Eli's original four cheesecakes into a dessert empire.

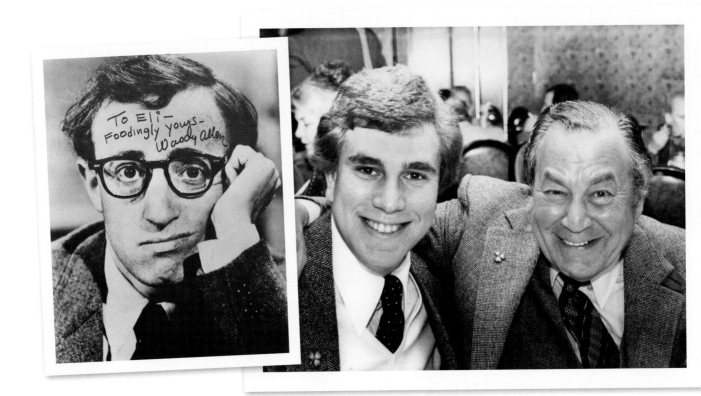

Eli's The Place For Steak

BY **MARC SCHULMAN**

PROVERB INSIDE MENU: *Great food always, at a profit if we can, at a loss if we must.*

"Love is the name of the game. I love people. Without people, I would be nobody. And my mother taught me, 'Charity will never bust you.'" —Eli Schulman

MY DAD, ELI SCHULMAN, WAS KNOWN AS THE SALAMI SURGEON DURING HIS DAYS AT ELI'S STAGE DELICATESSEN. The Deli was such a popular hangout among the singles of the '60s that my dad would often plop a parking meter on tables that had been occupied for too long. He'd gleefully announce "Your time is up!" once they overstayed their welcome. He could also be overheard telling the occasional lingering customer to "take it to go" as he transferred the contents of his or her coffee mug into a Styrofoam cup.

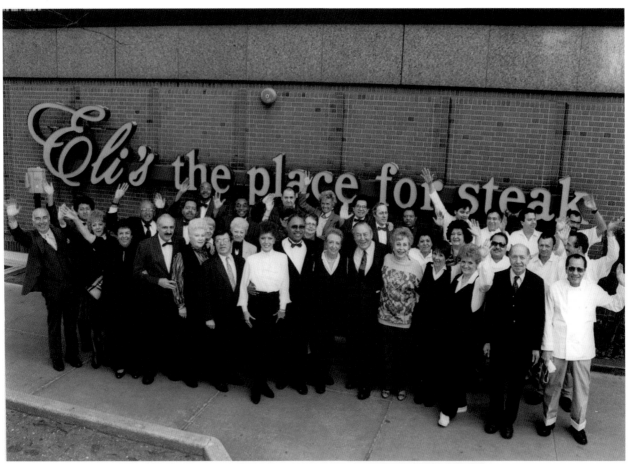

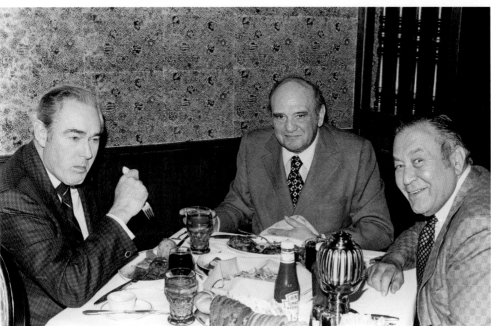

OPPOSITE, FROM LEFT: *Woody Allen loved to dine at Eli's when he was playing clubs in Chicago; law student Marc with Eli at the restaurant.*

ABOVE: *Class picture with Eli and Esther and the Eli's The Place For Steak team.*

LEFT: *Seen every Monday night at Table 30: President of the Cook County Board George Dunne and local politician Ira Colitz, in this photo joined by Eli. There were always others hoping to get some business done.*

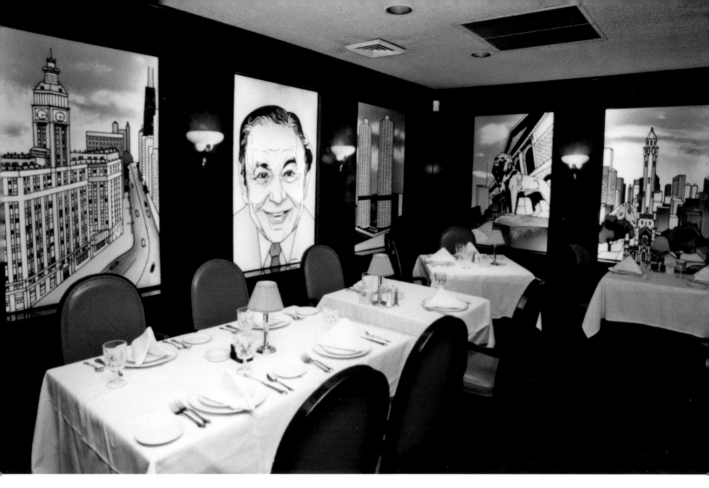

The interior of Eli's The Place For Steak, the first restaurant architect Martin Lescht ever designed.

Eli was always dreaming. He loved the Deli, but he also wanted to create a white-tablecloth restaurant that could take advantage of his deli roots—a steakhouse where he could also serve traditional Jewish favorites like chopped liver, potato pancakes, and chicken in the pot. He envisioned a place with ambiance and elegance, a place for his politician, celebrity, and athlete friends to gather and enjoy the very best steaks that Eli's dear friend, Bobby Hatoff of Stockyards Packing and later Allen Brothers Meats, had to offer.

In 1966, Eli's dream became a reality when Eli's The Place For Steak opened in the lobby of the Carriage House, an apartment hotel on Chicago Avenue just east of Michigan Avenue. For the critical role of maitre d', Eli recruited Monroe Elfenbein, who had been the host at Mr. Kelly's, a nightclub right down the street from the Deli, and was also a veteran of the Copacabana in New York. Eli kept the Deli open for several years while also running Eli's The Place For Steak, but eventually, a fire forced him to close, and he brought the Deli's staff over to the steakhouse.

Eli found that he liked having only one restaurant. He could greet every customer and give each the same individualized attention as he would a celebrity. That's exactly why he enforced a "jacket-required" dress code. "You never know if it's someone's birthday, and they only go out to dinner once a year," he'd say. I held my breath once, when the White Sox's manager, Jim Fregosi, came in wearing a very nice sweater. He was whisked off to the check room to choose a sport coat to wear during dinner. (Chances are, it was one of mine. Good thing he was tall.)

Eli used to work six days a week until one Sunday night, when Mayor Richard J. Daley arrived unannounced. "Eli here?" the first Mayor Daley asked. When the staff told him that he was off that night, the Mayor left without eating. After that, Eli added Sundays to his workweek.

Eli's The Place For Steak was like a club, a home away from home for its regulars—dark, comfortable, sheltered, with the kind of vibe that let you know deals were being made, secrets were being told, and Eli was at the helm.

Irv Kupcinet—known, of course, as Kup to everyone—was at Eli's The Place For Steak as often as three times a day. He'd appear first at lunch with his regular group, which included Chicago Bears Chairman Ed McCaskey, Steve Neal, Ray Coffey, fight promoter Ben Bentley, Howard Bedno, Sherman Wolf, and Jeremiah Joyce. Those lunches would stretch late into the afternoon, with Eli sneaking out to Arlington Park to catch his favorite horse, Eli's Cheesecake, in a race. Kup would return later with his wife, Essie, and join Eli and my mother, Esther, for dinner. Kup would surface again much later, when celebrities like Frank Sinatra were at Eli's The Place For Steak with Sammy Davis, Jr., Liza Minnelli, and their entourages.

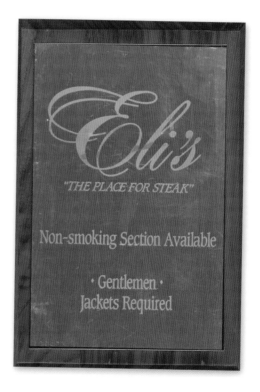

The plaque that hung by the entrance of the restaurant—jackets required.

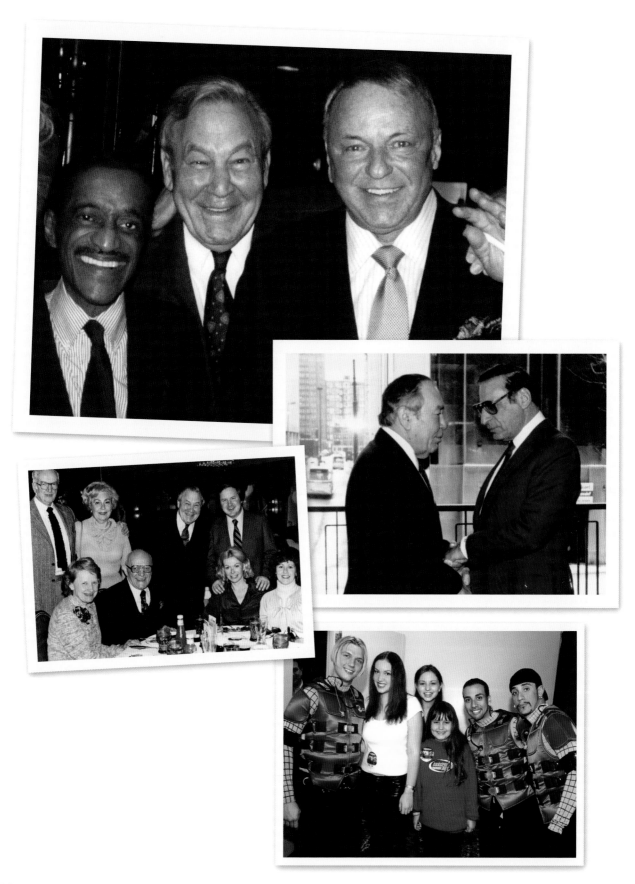

The regulars were there so often that the kitchen had a shelf set aside just for certain customers' favorites: Essie Kupcinet's hot sauce, a French press coffee pot for a couple who preferred plunged coffee, dry mustard for Cook County Board President George Dunne's mushroom salad with blue cheese (that wasn't on the menu), and white bread for when John Rogers ordered grilled cheese for dinner.

It's safe to say that Eli even launched a few political careers inside those four walls. Before he was elected Governor of Illinois, Eli's great friend James R. Thompson served as the United States Attorney for the Northern District of Illinois from 1971 to 1975. While in office, Thompson assembled a dream team of prosecutors who have gone on to great success in their careers, including Sam Skinner, Tony Valukas, Dan Webb, Ilana Rovner, Gary Starkman, and Joel Flaum, to name a few. Over the years, Thompson and his team frequently came to Eli's The Place For Steak for dinner after long days in the courtroom. Eli, always the consummate politician, made sure to seat defendants and their attorneys across the dining room from the prosecutors.

Eli and Thompson became close friends, and it was Eli who created Thompson's first political slogan on a button: "Big Jim Will Get the Job Done." When Eli presented the idea to Thompson one night at his table, Thompson quipped, "Eli, what's the job?" In 1975, Thompson successfully ran for governor and went on to hold the office for 14 years, making him the longest-serving governor in Illinois history.

Eli's The Place For Steak's piano bar, with legendary jazz and blues pianist Hal Roach at the keyboard, was a Chicago fixture. Roach knew all the regulars well and made a point of playing their favorite songs when they'd walk in. Maureen's was "Best That You

Sammy, Frank, and Eli: This was the first occasion that Sinatra visited Eli's The Place For Steak. Eli wasn't positive he was coming, but he'd heard rumors. That night, around 11:30 pm, the phone rang at Marc and Maureen's home. "He's here," Eli whispered; he wanted Maureen to come to the restaurant and take their picture. Maureen recalls: "We had two babies at home and no sitter, so we woke them up, got them dressed, and before long, found ourselves introducing them to the great Frank Sinatra. Turns out, he liked babies."

A common sight at The Place For Steak: Eli with Kup. Kup, who considered Eli to be one of his best sources, could often be found at Eli's as many as three times a day, entertaining and getting scoops.

Chicago Bears founder and legendary coach George "Papa Bear" Halas (seated, second from left) celebrated his birthday at Eli's with Esther and Eli Schulman (standing, second and third from left).

Eli's was a favorite of the Backstreet Boys. They dined there in 1999 during their Millennium Tour and again in 2005.

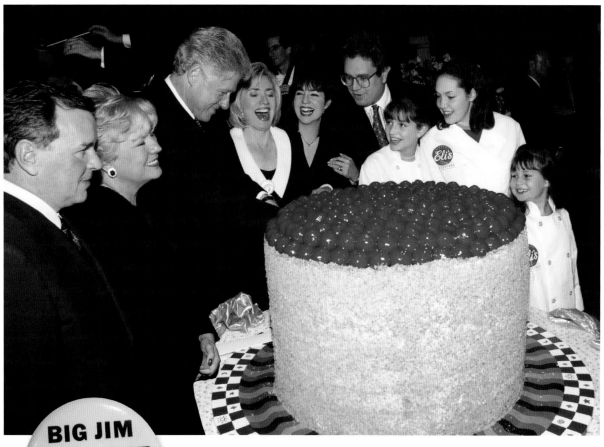

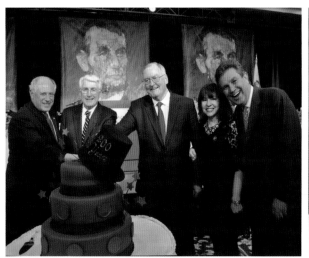

BIG JIM WILL GET THE JOB DONE

Then–First Lady Hillary Rodham Clinton celebrating her 50th birthday in Chicago. Surrounding her, left to right: Mayor Richard M. Daley and his wife, Maggie; President Bill Clinton; and Maureen, Marc, Kori, Haley, and Elana Schulman. The birthday cheesecake was a combination of Mrs. Clinton's favorite flavors: Eli's Chocolate Chip and Espresso Cheesecakes.

INSET: Jim Thompson's first political button, slogan courtesy of Eli Schulman (1975).

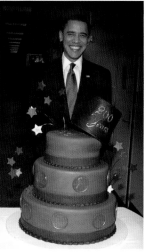

FROM LEFT: Past Illinois Governors Pat Quinn, Jim Edgar, and Jim Thompson with Maureen and Marc Schulman present a tiered chocolate cheesecake, decorated with edible copper-leafed chocolate pennies, for the celebration of Lincoln's bicentennial in Springfield, Illinois, in 2009.

President Barack Obama, a Lincoln aficionado, was the keynote speaker at the event.

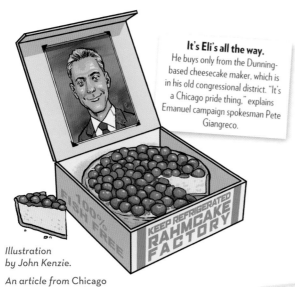

It's Eli's all the way.
He buys only from the Dunning-based cheesecake maker, which is in his old congressional district. "It's a Chicago pride thing," explains Emanuel campaign spokesman Pete Giangreco.

Illustration by John Kenzie.

An article from Chicago Magazine, September 2014.

RIGHT: *Bill Clinton visited Eli's Cheesecake during his first run for president. This photo ran on the front page of almost every major newspaper.*

BELOW: *Eli's was frequently asked to supply cheesecake to Air Force One, especially when the flight departed from Chicago. We were thrilled to receive this photo of President Clinton and Prime Minister of the United Kingdom Sir John Major being served Eli's Cheesecake on the plane.*

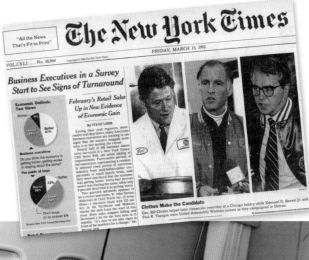

Eli (third from right) in 1982 with Chicago's business leaders and fellow McCormick Place board members at the opening of the first Morton's in Washington, DC.

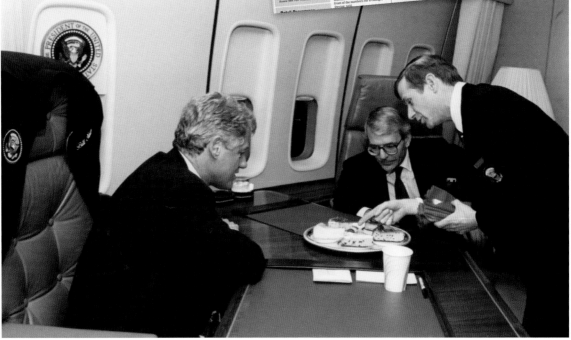

Can Do." Longtime society columnist Ann Gerber's was "Satin Doll." Hal always played "My Funny Valentine" for Merri Dee. "Zip-A-Dee-Doo-Dah" and "Chat-

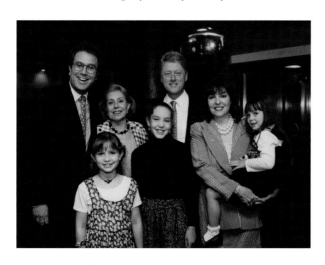

President Bill Clinton and the Schulman family at Eli's The Place For Steak.

tanooga Choo Choo" were our daughters' favorites, and they occasionally sang along with him at the bar.

The best entrance of all occurred one night when President Bill Clinton came to Eli's The Place For Steak for dinner. The Secret Service agents had warned me not to tell anyone, including the staff, of the President's impending arrival. Maureen suggested giving Hal a heads up not to react, but the agents flatly refused. Sure enough, when the President walked in, Hal looked up and without hesitation played a robust rendition of "Hail to the Chief." The secret was out.

In order to spend more time with my mother and me, my dad would close Eli's The Place For Steak on some of the biggest restaurant nights of the year: Mother's Day, Father's Day, and for three weeks over the Christmas holidays. My dad proudly passed on his Eli gems of wisdom, which taught me to respect the people I work with. His first rule was: "Treat the other as if you are the other." At Eli's The Place For Steak, the most valuable people were the busboys and the dishwashers—those who turned the tables and kept the dining room and kitchen pristine.

One of Eli's dearest friends was the late Steve Neal, political editor of the *Chicago Sun-Times.* Shortly after my dad passed away in May of 1988, Neal wrote: "Although Eli Schulman liked to get around, the town's great saloon keeper was a constant presence in his own place...Schulman would be working the table, greeting friends at the entrance of his dining room or sitting with some of the regulars in a chair with a good view of the door. Schulman never missed a detail...Eli Schulman was a great and good man."

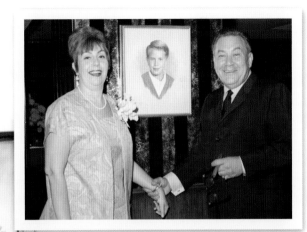

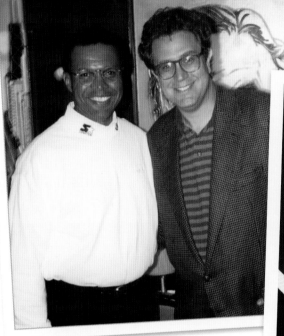

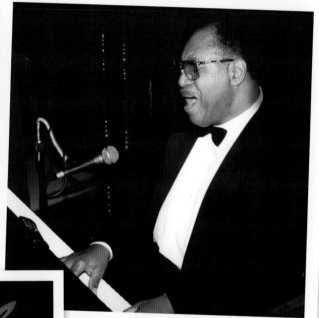

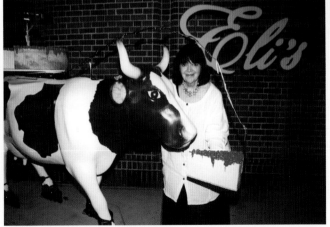

CLOCKWISE FROM TOP RIGHT:

Esther and Eli with a photo of Marc on the wall at the Eli's entryway.

Legendary piano bar entertainer Hal Roach tickled the ivories at Eli's for more than 36 years.

Second City producer Joyce Sloane, known as the "mother of Chicago theater," with Eli's "Cows on Parade" sculpture.

Chicago Bears football great Gale Sayers, a very close friend of Eli Schulman, poses at the restaurant with Marc.

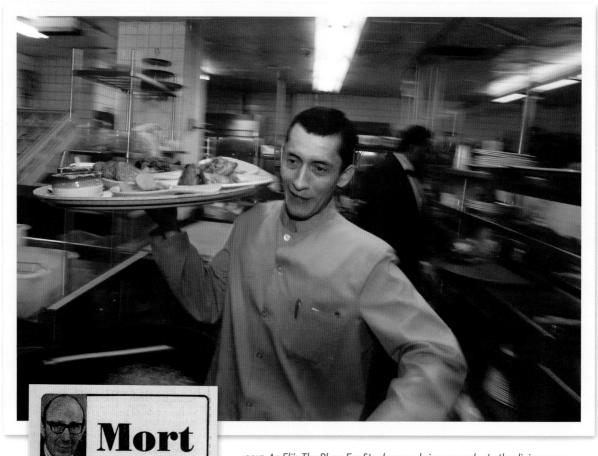

ABOVE: *An Eli's The Place For Steak server brings an order to the dining room.*

LEFT: *Tony Martin and Cyd Charisse at Eli's.*

Mort

By Mort Edelstein

THAT WAS **Tony Martin** and his lovely wife, **Cyd Charisse**, in Eli's Place for steak, talking about the old days when he played the Chez Paree in Chicago. Tony, starring with Cyd in the Empire Room, was a longtime favorite of Chez Paree, audiences when the club was owned by **Mike Fritzel** and **Joey Jacobson**. One of Martin's best friends in Chicago is real estate tycoon **Aaron Weiner**.

OPPOSITE, CLOCKWISE FROM TOP:

Two cooks prepare Liver Eli in the restaurant's kitchen.

There were always so many celebs at Eli's that this columnist called the restaurant a "swingin' pad."

Bears Coach Jim Dooley and Jack Benny dining at Eli's.

Dinah Shore at Eli's.

CHICAGO SUN-TIMES,   MONDAY, SEPTEMBER 26, 1994

Celebs
By Bill Zwecker

Eli's Pianist Keys Clinton Arrival

President Clinton got his just desserts Friday. After attending the big Democratic Senatorial Campaign fund-raiser at the Ritz-Carlton, the prez made a beeline for Eli's The Place for Steak, where the Secret Service told owner **Marc Schulman** "to keep it low key."

Yeah, like *no one* would notice the president of the United States dropping by. Sworn to secrecy, Schulman and his wife, **Maureen**, didn't tell any staff members about Clinton's arrival. But **Hal Roach**, Eli's legendary piano player, didn't miss a beat. Even though he had no idea the president was expected, he started playing "Hail to the Chief" as soon as he spied Clinton crossing the threshold.

"So much for keeping it low key," quipped Schulman. "As soon as Hal started playing, everyone in the entire restaurant stood up with their mouths hanging open!"

Joined by **Bill Daley, David Wilhelm, Tom Hynes** and **Tom Lyons,** Clinton shook hands with diners before sitting down to dessert and coffee. On his plate: a half-slice each of original plain Eli's cheesecake and their new apple tart.

ZONING ZINGER: A spokeswoman for the Long Island town of Southampton, N.Y., confirms that the guest house in which tennis star **Vitas Gerulaitis** died was *not* zoned for residential use. It was zoned as a pool house, having far less stringent building code requirements, since people are not expected to live in it. The pool house is part of the complex owned by **Martin and Patty Raynes.** She's the daughter of entertainment mogul and oil man **Marvin Davis,** and sources say the Rayneses had long fought with Southampton authorities over zoning issues while building their elaborate mansion. ■ Though representatives for Gerulaitis' estate refused to comment, other sources claim that a major lawsuit is being prepped charging negligence. Gerulaitis was asphyxiated because of faulty gas heating equipment.

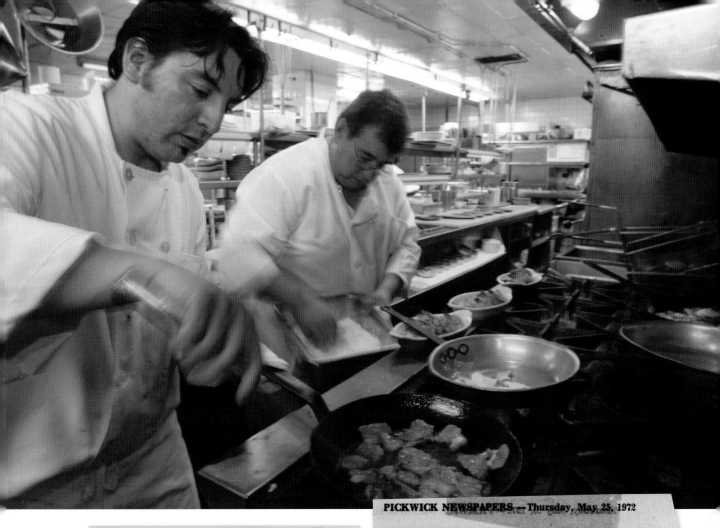

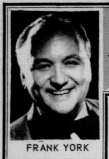

In his book *Unforgettable*, Scott Simon recalled, "Eli's The Place For Steak was a 'watering hole' for athletes, celebs and pols who liked to see their names in bold letters in tabloid columns the next day. The era of Eli's was the time of Irv Kupcinet (aka Kup), the legendary columnist for the *Chicago Sun-Times* who wrote for almost 60 years."

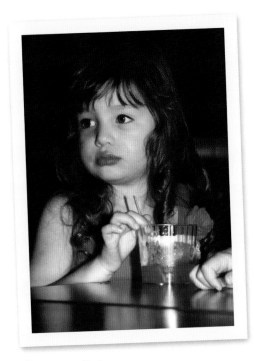

Kori enjoys a Shirley Temple at the bar.

For me, The Place For Steak was truly home. I met my wife, Maureen, when she was a customer at Table 10. I lived above the store, so to speak, while I was in law school at Northwestern. My dad loved it—he would call me every night to come down and meet someone interesting who had come in for dinner. We even stopped at Eli's The Place For Steak before bringing each of our newborn daughters home from the hospital. My family and I celebrated every holiday and special occasion at the restaurant, from the time I was eleven years old until it closed in 2005 to make way for the construction of the Ann and Robert H. Lurie Children's Hospital of Chicago. When our now-not-so-little girl Kori was two years old, we'd often ask her on warm, sunny days whether she'd like to play in the park or visit with my dad in the bar. She'd always pick the bar.

I was fortunate that my dad's greatest creation was his signature cheesecake, because unfortunately, liver just doesn't have the same universal appeal. Yet I regularly get approached by former customers of Eli's The Place For Steak who ask, "When will you reopen?" They miss the dishes that Eli's was famous for, and that's the inspiration for this chapter of the cookbook. Put on your favorite Sinatra song, have a martini, and enjoy these great dishes at home.

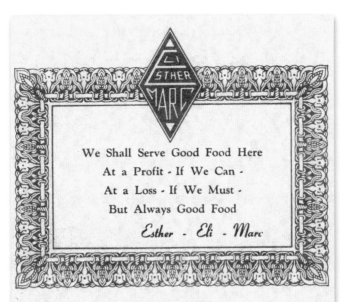

We Shall Serve Good Food Here
At a Profit - If We Can -
At a Loss - If We Must -
But Always Good Food

Esther - Eli - Marc

Eli's The Place For Steak
menu cover, circa 1978,
features Eli's mantra:
"Good food always..."

Appeteasers and Soups

French Onion Soup Baked in Crock, au Gratin **2.00**

Jumbo Shrimp a la Marc **4.00** Jumbo Shrimp Cocktail, Tangy Sauce **4.00**
Filets of Herring, Sour Cream **2.00** Chopped Chicken Livers **2.00**
Shrimp de Jonghe **4.00** Bar-B-Q Rib Appetizer **3.50**

Breaded Boneless Breast of Chicken Cutlet
Sauteed Mushrooms, Creamed Broccoli "A Real Treat" **9.45**

Broiled Calves Liver Steak Fresh Genuine Calves Liver
Cut Like a Sirloin and Broiled to Taste, Sure to Please **9.45**

T-Bone Steak 20 oz.
Broiled to your taste, for those hearty eaters **15.45**

Choice of Salad and Potatoes

Potatoe Skins **Onion Rings**
Apple Sauce or Sour Cream **2.50**
1.00

Entrees of Distinction

CALVES LIVER, ELI
Tops in Quality - Tops in Freshness - Tops in Taste
Sliced Calves Liver Sauteed with Onions, Green Peppers and
Mushrooms "Don't Hesitate" Delicious **9.45**

BREADED VEAL CUTLET
Tender Veal, Breaded and Delicately Seasoned
Tomato Sauce **8.95**

ELI'S SPECIAL SIRLOIN STEAK
Charred and Seasoned with Ground Pepper Corns
To Please the Spicy Taste Buds **13.95**

Roast Prime Native Rib Eye of Beef, Natural au Jus
A Thick Eye Cut of Corn Fed Prime Beef at its Finest **10.95**

Tournedos of Prime Beef Tenderloin Brown Butter Saute,
Twin Center Cuts of Succulent Tenderloin **11.95**

Broiled Chopped Steak, Esther
Freshly Chopped Sirloin, Made from a Recipe Handed Down Thru the
Years That Brings Out That Old World Flavor "A Must" **8.45**

Italian Pepper Steak Sauce au Vin Rouge, Sliced Tenderloin of Beef,
Mushrooms, Tomatoes and Green Peppers in Wine Sauce **11.95**

The Ladies Steak a la Mignon
For the More Petit Appetite, Prime Center Cut Beef Tenderloin, Broiled to Her Taste **10.95**

Salads
Thinly Sliced Tomatoes and Bermuda Onions **2.50** Fresh Spinach & Mushroom Salad **2.50**

Desserts and Beverages
Brandy Ice **2.00** Irish Coffee **2.00** Esther's Special Cheese Cake **1.75**
Fresh Fruit in Season **1.50** French Ice Cream or Sherbet **1.25**

*In Chicago
"for Good Food"
it's Eli's*

Entrees of the Open Hearth Broiler

Bar-B-Que Genuine Canadian Baby Back Ribs
A Whole Slab of Tender Ribs, Smoked in the
Old Fashioned Way **9.45**

Prime Sirloin Steak Delmonico
Served with a Tangy Sauce **12.95**

Old Fashioned Hamburger Patties a la Essie
Years Ago They Called Them Cutletten, Now the Same Old Flavor
with a New Name **8.45**

Filet Mignon of Beef Tenderloin (Prime Center Cut)
A Borrowed French Idea, Magnificently Portrayed by
Prime Native Beef Tenderloin **12.95**

Top of the Sirloin Butt Steak (Center Cut)
Open Hearth Broiled, Crisp Onion Rings **9.95**

Broiled Jr. N.Y. Strip Sirloin Steak
Tender and Delicious **12.95**

Broiled Fancy French Cut Double Lamb Chops
Extra Thick, Prime Loin Lamb Chops, Mint Jelly **12.95**

Broiled New York Cut Strip Sirloin Steak Mushroom Cap,
Our Finest Steak, This is Truly the King of all Steaks **13.95**

Chateaubriand Le Bearnaise (for two)
A Full Center Cut Tenderloin Filet That Truly Fits the Bill for any
Special Occasion with Vegetable Bouquetiere **26.00**

From the Briney Deep and Inland Seas

Broiled Filet of Fresh Lake Superior Whitefish
A Firm White Meat Filet Seasoned to
Perfection, Lemon Butter **9.45**

Filet of Imported Dover Sole
This Delicious Fish is caught off The "White Cliffs
of Dover" in The English Channel, Almondine,
Boned Delicately **12.95**

Baked Shrimp De Jonghe Served en Casserole,
A Chicago Original, Jumbo Gulf Shrimps, Simmered in Wine and Broiled
with Zesty Garlic Butter **9.45**

Fresh Boston Scrod
Eli's Newest Specialty **8.45**

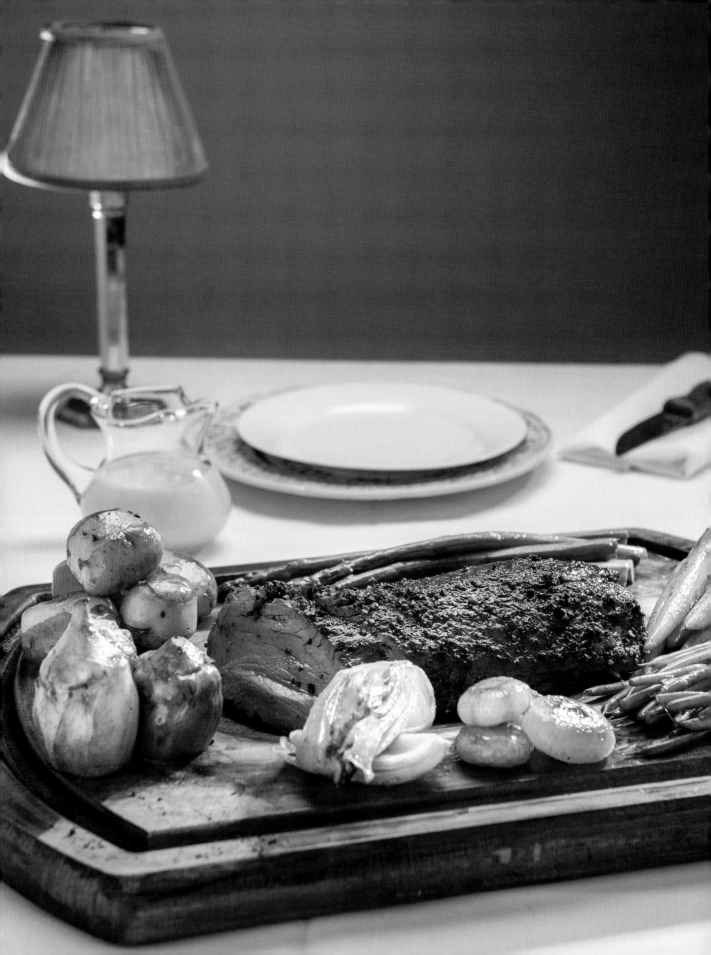

Chateaubriand

YIELD: 4-5 ENTRÉE SERVINGS

Eli bought all of his custom-cut, dry-aged meats from his close friend Bobby Hatoff, a meat purveyor who was first with Stockyards Packing and later moved on to Allen Brothers. Our family always ordered the Chateaubriand for special occasions, birthdays, and anniversaries. It was prepared perfectly, tender on the inside but beautifully charred on the outside, and served with a colorful array of vegetables. Today, I make beef tenderloin for every special occasion at home.

¼ cup black peppercorns, cracked

2½ pounds beef tenderloin, center cut trimmed

1 teaspoon vegetable oil

Water, for blanching

1-2 teaspoons salt, for blanching

1 medium bunch asparagus, trimmed

6 ounces green beans

8 whole small new red potatoes

3 whole baby artichokes

8 ounces cipollini onions, sliced

8-10 ounces baby carrots, sliced

1 large bulb fennel, sliced

2 tablespoons unsalted butter

1. Rub the cracked black peppercorns all over the beef, ensuring that the entire surface of the meat is covered. Cover and chill overnight in the refrigerator.

2. Set the oven rack at the middle position and preheat the oven to 325°F. Remove the beef from the refrigerator.

3. Warm a large cast iron skillet over medium–high heat until a drop of water dances on the skillet's surface. Then, using a paper towel or brush, coat the skillet's surface with the oil. Immediately place the beef in the center of the skillet and sear it, rotating it often, until all surfaces of the meat are browned. (Note: You will know the meat is adequately browned when it lifts off the skillet easily.)

4. Transfer the meat to the center rack of the oven and cook for about 30 to 35 minutes, until the meat's internal temperature reaches 120°F for medium rare.

RECIPE CONTINUES ON PAGE 46

CHATEAUBRIAND (CONTINUED FROM PAGE 45)

5. *Blanch the vegetables:* Place a large saucepan filled halfway with water over medium–high heat. Place a large bowl filled with ice water next to the cooktop. Once the water is boiling, plunge the asparagus into it and allow to boil for 2 minutes. Using a slotted spoon, remove the asparagus from the saucepan and plunge it into the ice bath. Taste for doneness, and if satisfied, transfer the asparagus to a strainer to drain. If not, return to the boiling water and repeat each minute until the appropriate level of doneness is reached. Repeat with the remaining vegetables, one at a time. Remove from the heat.

6. Remove the skillet from the oven and tent with foil, allowing the meat to rest for 15 minutes before slicing.

7. While the meat is resting, warm the butter in a nonstick skillet over medium heat. Add the blanched vegetables and sauté for 2 to 3 minutes, stirring occasionally. Remove from the heat.

8. Slice the meat and arrange it on a platter with the sautéed vegetables. Serve family style.

46 *THE ELI'S CHEESECAKE COOKBOOK*

Liver Eli

YIELD: 4 ENTRÉE SERVINGS

Liver Eli has long been credited with turning liver haters into liver lovers. In a 1988 interview with Sun-Times *columnist Bob Herguth, Eli recalled how he developed the famous recipe: "Remember how your mother made good things? I was at a club in Florida and ordered liver. The way it was described on the menu, it reminded me of my mother's. When the liver arrived, I didn't like it. I decided to recreate dishes that came from old recipes, the kind our mothers made."*

If a customer seemed hesitant about ordering liver, Eli would send a steak appetizer to the table, on the house. Once they'd raved about how good it was, he'd spring the truth on them: Surprise! It had been Liver Eli all along!

One person who didn't need convincing was Marlene Siskel, wife of the late film critic Gene Siskel. She recalled that strolling into Eli's The Place For Steak was "like walking into an era when Chicago was Sinatra's kind of town. For me, it was Eli's The Place For Liver. I had never eaten liver before, nor have I since the restaurant closed. It was that good, and I didn't want to cloud the memory of its incredible taste and texture by ordering it anywhere else."

1 pound fresh calves liver, veins and membrane removed

1½ cups whole milk

⅓ cup all-purpose flour

½ teaspoon salt

½ teaspoon freshly ground black pepper

4–6 tablespoons vegetable oil, divided

5 medium red, yellow, or green peppers, cut into 1½-inch squares

1 large Spanish onion, peeled and sliced lengthwise

⅓ teaspoon sweet paprika

5 tablespoons unsalted butter

1 clove garlic, minced

3 tablespoons beef broth

3 tablespoons dry white wine

3 tablespoons chopped parsley, for garnish (optional)

RECIPE CONTINUES ON PAGE 48

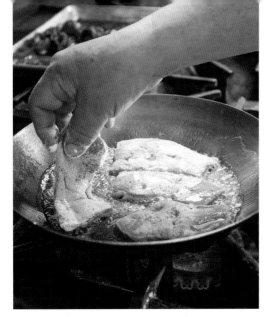

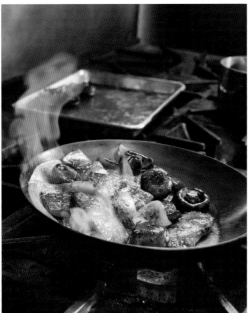

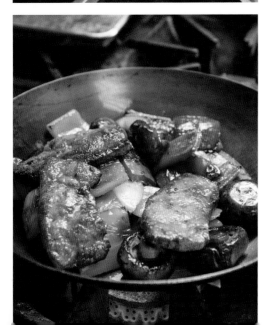

LIVER ELI *(CONTINUED FROM PAGE 47)*

1. Cut the liver diagonally into ¼-inch slices. Place in a ceramic or glass bowl and cover with the milk. Cover and chill in the refrigerator for at least 3 hours.

2. In a small bowl, mix together the flour, salt, and pepper. Sprinkle the mixture evenly onto a large, flat platter.

3. Drain the liver slices, discarding the milk. Using paper towels, pat the slices dry and transfer them to a wire rack.

4. In a large, heavy-bottomed skillet over medium–high heat, warm 3 tablespoons of the oil. Add the peppers to the skillet, skin side down, and fry, turning once, for 3 to 4 minutes, until the peppers are softened and browned around the edges. Using a slotted spoon, transfer the peppers to a platter lined with a paper towel to drain any excess oil.

5. Add the onions to the skillet (along with another tablespoon of the oil, if necessary) and sauté for 4 to 5 minutes, until the onions are golden brown and softened, but not limp. Transfer the onions to the lined platter and sprinkle the paprika over the vegetables.

6. Reduce the heat to medium and add 1 tablespoon of the oil and the butter to the skillet. When the oil and butter begins to shimmer, quickly dip both sides of the liver pieces into the flour mixture. Shaking off the excess flour, place the slices, one at a time, into the hot skillet. Carefully avoid crowding the pieces in the skillet. Fry each slice for 6 seconds on each side, until it begins to brown around the edges. As each slice is sufficiently cooked, transfer it to a platter tented with foil. Repeat, adding oil as needed, until all slices of the liver are cooked.

7. Add the garlic to the skillet and sauté for 1 minute. Add the beef stock and wine to the skillet and simmer for 8 to 10 minutes, until the liquid has reduced by half.

8. Return the vegetables and liver to the skillet and warm through. Remove from the heat. Transfer to a platter and serve hot. Garnish with the chopped parsley, if desired.

---

10   CHICAGO SUN-TIMES, Mon., Sept. 5, 1977

Eli, who turned the high-livers into liver-lovers

By F. K. Plous Jr.

Usually it takes only a couple of words to sum up a person's life: Doctor or merchant or musician. Parent or celebrity or churchgoer. Nice guy or bum.

But try to pin a label on Eli Schulman, the bouncing Jewish leprechaun who runs Eli's, the Place for Steak, at 215 E. Chicago, and you'll find it's not that simple.

Schulman, at 61, has too big a dossier. He rose from the poverty of a West Side ghetto in the Depression to become one of the city's top restaurateurs; he was a Democratic precinct captain at 20 and stayed one for 25 years; he rubs shoulders nightly with movie stars, athletes, surgeons, federal judges and governors. He has given away small fortunes to charity and persuaded others to do the same; he's a high school dropout, but students in Israel, 6,000 miles away, thank him for helping them complete their education, and graduate students at De Paul University fill lecture halls to hear him speak.

But the man who chisels the epitaph into Schulman's tombstone will probably immortalize an even more difficult accomplishment. Don't be surprised if the stone reads:

"Eli Schulman, 1916 — : "He made 'em eat liver and love it."

It's true. Hundreds of well heeled regulars who patronize Schulman's restaurant routinely bypass the renowned steaks, ribs, chops and seafood to dine on a plate of humble calves' liver with onions and green peppers.

"Joe DiMaggio comes in here and all he orders is that liver," Schulman beamed. "Chef Louis Szathmary from the Bakery comes in here for the liver, and he sends his friends here and tells THEM they have to have the liver. I have had people in here who say, 'If you put a gun to my head I won't touch liver.' And those same people bring their friends in and beg 'em to taste it."

It's the philosophy behind the recipe that makes the dish successful, and Schulman uses the same philosophy on the customers: care, patience, lots of personal attention. He says he used the same philosophy when he started his first restaurant, the Ogden Huddle, at Ogden and Kedzie, in 1941.

"I opened up just before the war," he said.

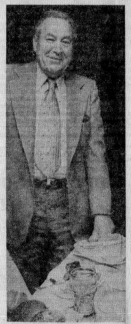

ELI SCHULMAN—he makes 'em eat liver and love it. (Sun-Times Photo by Chuck Kirman)

"On Pearl Harbor day I thought I ought to do something, so I put a coupla signs in the window. One said, 'If you are hungry and have no

CITYSCAPE

money, come in and we'll feed you free.' The other one said, '25-per cent discount for men and women in uniform.' "

It was the start of something Schulman has continued throughout his career — giving. True, donating to charity has been long a tradition among Jewish businessmen, especially the prominent. The difference with Schulman is that he started giving it away before he had very much of it and long before he was prominent.

"I was in the premium business once," he said, "and I still keep little prizes around in my office—radios, ashtrays, ball-point pens and that stuff. I like to give 'em away. You don't do things 'cause you want something out of it. You do it for the thrill of it. My mother taught me, 'Charity will never bust you.' "

Fortunately for a man of Schulman's habits, she taught him to make money as well as get rid of it. And she taught him just in time.

"When I opened my restaurant in 1941, I had never cracked an egg in my life," Schulman said. "Little did I know that necessity is the mother of invention. Four days later the cook didn't show.

"My first order was breaded veal cutlet. I didn't know the difference between beef, veal and pork, so I called my mother on the phone. She told me in her half-Jewish, half-English brogue what to do, and I cooked it, and the guy who ordered it said it was great. Two days later I got a new cook and the guy came in again and ordered veal cutlet. He said it wasn't as good as the last time."

That sort of thing can give a man the impression he's made for the restaurant business, and as soon as Schulman returned from the Army he jumped right back in. First it was a grill at Argyle and Sheridan, followed in the late '50s by Eli's Stage Delicatessen on Oak St. Business on Oak St. was slow for a while, but it seemed to skyrocket mysteri-

ously in the early '60s right after Schulman threw a free Passover seder for some Jewish singles who had no place else to celebrate the traditional meal.

"I was gonna charge 'em $5 apiece," Schulman said, "and when I saw how much they were eating I decided to raise it to $10. Then I thought: What's Passover? It's when you share with a stranger. I didn't charge 'em anything. Business improved right after that."

In 1966, the big break came: Schulman made a deal to open a real steak house in the Carriage House Hotel. His habit of visiting personally at each table during the middle of the meal quickly won him the friendship of the famous, who were already getting addicted to the food. County Board President George W. Dunne became a regular. Ed McCaskey, vice president of the Chicago Bears, was hooked, and so were the Bears themselves, in particular Gale Sayers and the late Brian Piccolo. Later, when Piccolo was dying of cancer in New York, Schulman flew to see him.

Success meant more than a higher income and famous friends to Schulman. It meant he could give on a scale he had never imagined before. He picked a favorite charity — Community Assistance for Secondary Education. The organization channels money into scholarships for Israeli students who cannot afford a high school education. Schulman gave thousands and signed up others for more thousands. The givers don't seem to resent his appeals for assistance, either. On Sunday, they're scheduled to gather in the grand ballroom of the Conrad Hilton to thank Schulman publicly at a testimonial banquet.

The dinner and the speeches will formalize at last what hundreds of Chicagoans have known for more than a decade: Eli Schulman is one of the few people who in the span of one lifetime made the transition from ghetto hustler to philanthropist. It was a difficult task, but it can't possibly have been as hard as it was to get all those celebrities to enjoy liver.

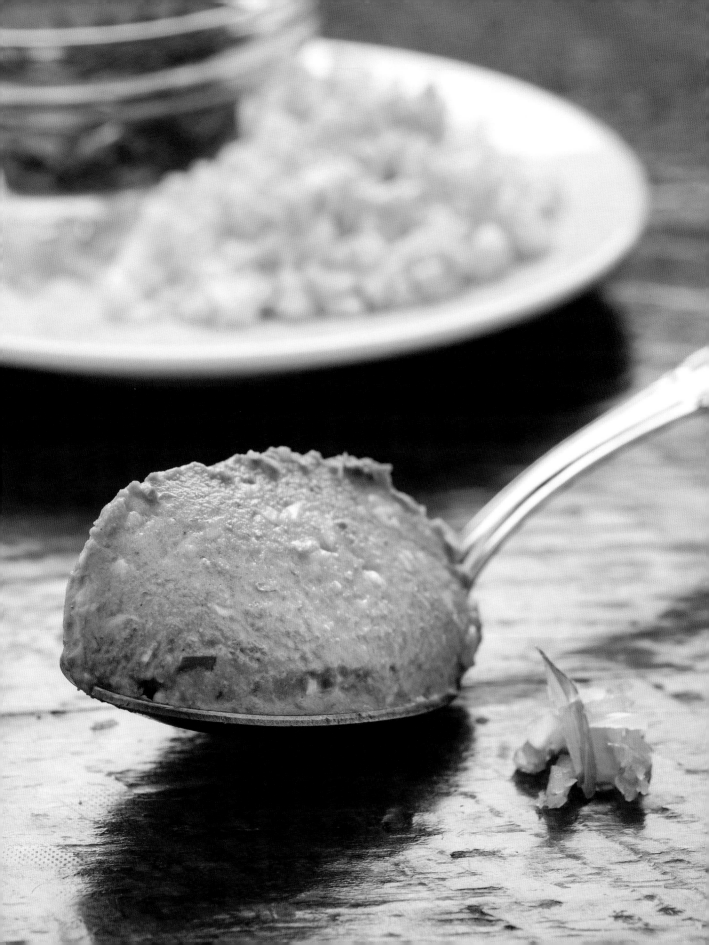

Chopped Liver Eli

YIELD: 8-10 APPETIZER SERVINGS

Over the years, Eli's The Place For Steak won numerous "Best Bread Basket" awards from local publications. Immediately after being seated, patrons were greeted by a busboy carrying a chilled dish of crudités, a bread basket overflowing with matzoh and raisin pumpernickel bread (which Eli had delivered daily via cab from Kaufman's, a Jewish bakery on the North Side), and an oval platter heaped with chopped liver, eggs, and onion. Although Eli's The Place For Steak has closed, you can still enjoy one of Eli's favorites!

¼ cup olive oil, divided
1 large Spanish onion, finely chopped
1 pound chicken livers, trimmed and patted dry
Salt and freshly ground black pepper, to taste
6 large whole eggs, hard boiled and peeled
1-2 tablespoons water (optional)

1. In a heavy-bottomed skillet over medium heat, warm 2 tablespoons of the oil. Add the onion and sauté, stirring occasionally, for 4 to 5 minutes, until golden brown. Transfer to a bowl.

2. Add the chicken livers and the remaining 2 tablespoons of oil to the skillet and sear, turning once, for 3 minutes. Reduce the heat to medium and continue to cook for 3 minutes, until firm. Remove from the heat and transfer to a plate. Sprinkle with the salt and pepper and set aside to cool to room temperature.

3. In the bowl of a food processor fitted with the "S" blade, combine the eggs and sautéed onion. Pulse the mixture until it is well blended and finely chopped. Transfer to a mixing bowl.

4. Place the livers in the food processor bowl and pulse until they are finely chopped. Add the livers to the egg–onion mixture and stir until well combined. Season with the salt and pepper. If the mixture is too crumbly, add as much of the water as you need to moisten it. Serve with matzoh, bread, and a relish tray.

Shrimp à la Marc

YIELD: 4 APPETIZER SERVINGS

Eli's The Place For Steak was well known for this delicious appetizer: Chilled, fresh shrimp marinated in a tangy mix of sour cream, onions, and capers. Eli loved it so much, he named it after his only son. The connection paid off for Marc, too—during an interview with a prestigious law firm, Marc waited anxiously while the attorney interviewing him carefully perused his resume, wondering which of his many impressive achievements had captured the attorney's attention. But he had only one question: "Are you Shrimp Marc?"

1 medium Vidalia onion, thinly sliced

1 quart ice water

2 cups mayonnaise

1 cup sour cream, room temperature

1 tablespoon fresh lemon juice

½ teaspoon salt

1 pinch white pepper

2 drops Tabasco sauce

24 extra large whole cooked shrimp, peeled and deveined

1 tablespoon small capers, drained, plus more if desired

Salad greens, for garnish

1. Refresh the onion by submerging it in the water for 1 hour. Drain the onion and discard the water. Pat the onion dry with paper towels.

2. In a large mixing bowl, combine the mayonnaise, sour cream, lemon juice, salt, pepper, and Tabasco. Add the onions and stir until combined. Add the shrimp and capers and stir until combined. Chill in the refrigerator for at least 3 hours.

3. On chilled individual serving plates garnished with the greens, evenly arrange the shrimp with dollops of the mayonnaise sauce. Garnish with the additional capers, if desired, and serve.

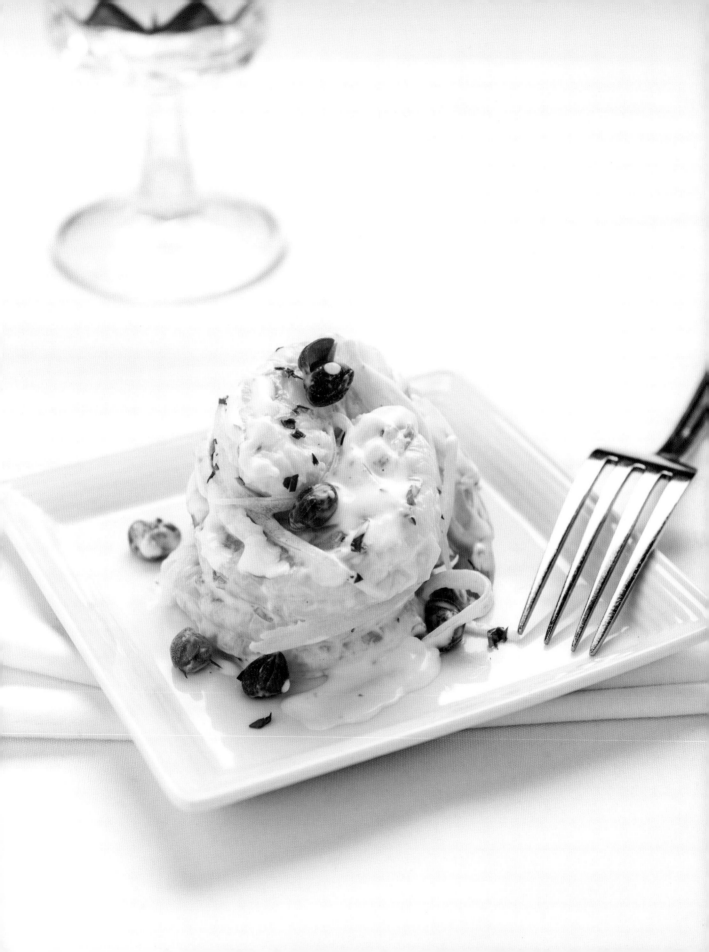

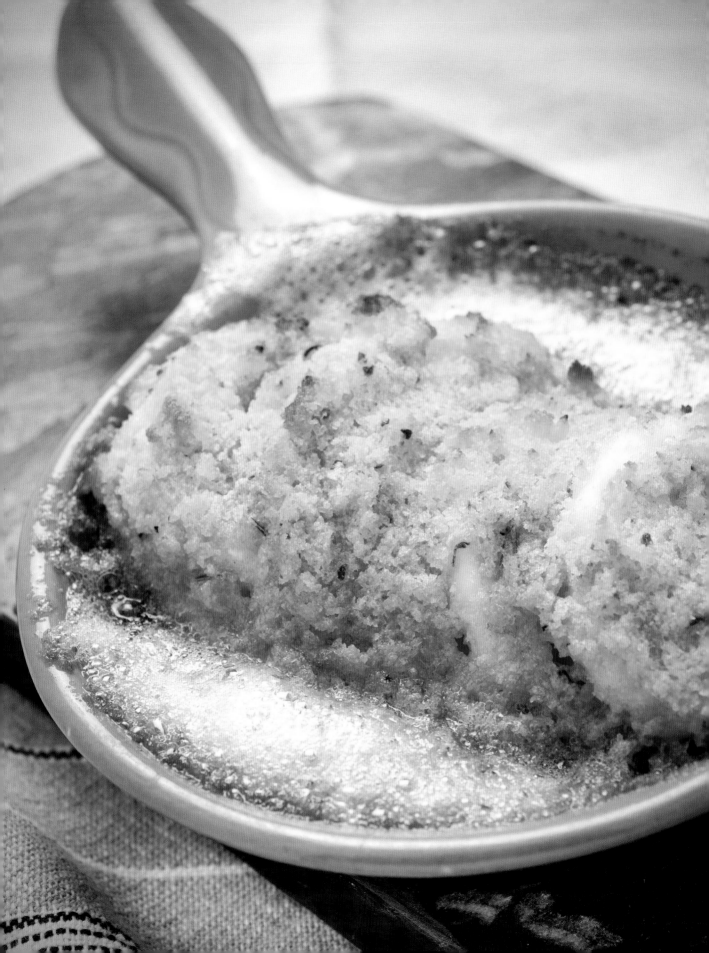

Shrimp de Jonghe

YIELD: 6 APPETIZER SERVINGS

"Eli's menu has a number of dishes born in Chicago, the most famous being Shrimp de Jonghe."
—Chicago Sun-Times *writer Pat Bruno*

Belgian brothers Henri, Pierre, and Charles de Jonghe owned a restaurant and hotel at 21 E. Monroe Street from the turn of the 20th century until it was closed by police following a Prohibition raid in 1923. Either the brothers or their chef, Emil Zehr, are responsible for the invention of a true Chicago classic, Shrimp de Jonghe. This super-garlicky, oozing with butter, crunchy breadcrumb-topped dish sold so well at Eli's The Place For Steak that the kitchen made 50 pounds of its Savory Butter Bread-crumb Crust a day.

"Eli's follows the original masterful creation closely. With my order, under a blanket of seasoned breadcrumbs, a lot of good shrimp came to know melted butter and an intense garlic flavor quite well. It was enough to make me believe that the de Jonghe brothers would have been most approving."
—*Pat Bruno,* Chicago Sun-Times, *April 5, 1992.*

1 pound cooked extra-large (26 to 30 count) shrimp, shell-on, rinsed
¼ cup white wine
1 recipe Savory Butter Breadcrumb Crust, chilled for 1 hour (recipe follows)

1. Preheat the oven to 375°F and adjust the rack so it is in the center of the oven. Arrange 6 (6-inch) ungreased shallow, ovenproof gratin dishes on a large baking sheet.

2. Divide and slightly mound 4 to 5 shrimp in the bottom of each gratin dish. Drizzle 1 tablespoon of the wine over each of the mounds of shrimp.

3. Slice the Savory Butter Breadcrumb Crust log into ¼-inch rounds. Place several of the sliced rounds, overlapping them slightly, on top of each of the mounds of shrimp, until they resemble the top of a pie crust.

4. Place the baking sheet on the center rack of the oven and bake for 10 to 12 minutes, until the crust is browned. Remove from the oven and serve hot in the gratin dishes.

NOTE: Making this recipe means you'll witness a culinary miracle! The pastry-like Savory Butter Breadcrumb Crust bathes the shrimp in melted butter as it cooks, which simultaneously steams the shrimp, bastes it, and seasons it.

Savory Butter Breadcrumb Crust

YIELD: 1 CRUST FOR SHRIMP DE JONGHE

1½ cups salted butter, room temperature

2 tablespoons shallots, minced

2 teaspoons minced garlic

3 tablespoons minced fresh Italian parsley

1 teaspoon Worcestershire sauce

2 drops chili sauce

¼ teaspoon celery salt

4 cups lightly toasted coarse bread crumbs

1. In a large mixing bowl, combine the butter, shallots, garlic, parsley, Worcestershire sauce, chili sauce, and celery salt. Stir until well combined. Add the bread crumbs and stir until just combined.

2. Transfer the mixture to a cutting board and form it into a 2-inch × 12-inch log. Wrap the log in parchment paper and chill in the refrigerator for 2 hours, until firm.

Chicken in the Pot with Matzoh Balls

YIELD: 2 SERVINGS

Eli's The Place For Steak's regulars were addicted to Eli's Chicken in the Pot, especially during long Chicago winters. Our very own Jewish penicillin started with a huge bowl of golden broth that was really flavorful, yet never too salty. It had plenty of vegetables, tender boiled chicken, and delicate, not heavy, matzoh balls. It was listed as Haley's favorite, for our oldest daughter, who ordered it all the time. Our family celebrated every holiday at Eli's, and Chicken in the Pot was always on the menu.

1–2 tablespoons salt

1 3-pound fresh broiler/fryer chicken, skin on and cut into 4 pieces

2½ quarts chicken stock (preferably homemade)

1 small carrot, diced

3 stalks celery, diced

½ small Spanish onion, diced

1 small bay leaf

5 whole peppercorns

1 stem fresh Italian parsley

1 recipe Matzoh Balls (recipe on p. 58)

1. To a 4-quart pot ¾ full of water over medium heat, add the salt and chicken. Cook for 35 to 40 minutes, until it almost reaches a simmer and a meat thermometer inserted in one of the chicken thighs registers 160°F. Remove from the heat. Using tongs, remove the chicken from the pot and place it in a bowl. Discard the water and clean the pot.

2. Carefully rinse the chicken, removing all scum, and return it to the clean pot. Add the chicken stock, carrot, celery, onion, bay leaf, and peppercorns to the pot and place it over medium–high heat. Cover the pot and poach the chicken for 10 minutes, until hot.

3. Add the Matzoh Balls to the pot and bring to a simmer. Remove from the heat, transfer to bowls, and serve hot.

Matzoh Balls

YIELD: 2 SERVINGS

4 quarts water

1/3 teaspoon salt

1/4 teaspoon white pepper

1 cup matzoh meal

4 large whole eggs, room temperature

3/4 cup chicken stock

1/4 cup chicken fat

1. In a large pot over medium–high heat, bring the water to a boil and add the salt and pepper.

2. In a large bowl, mix together the matzoh meal, eggs, stock, and fat. Stir until well combined.

3. Using a 2-inch ice cream scoop, form the mixture into balls. Gently drop each matzoh ball into the boiling water and poach them for 5 minutes, until they float to the surface. Remove from the pot and set aside.

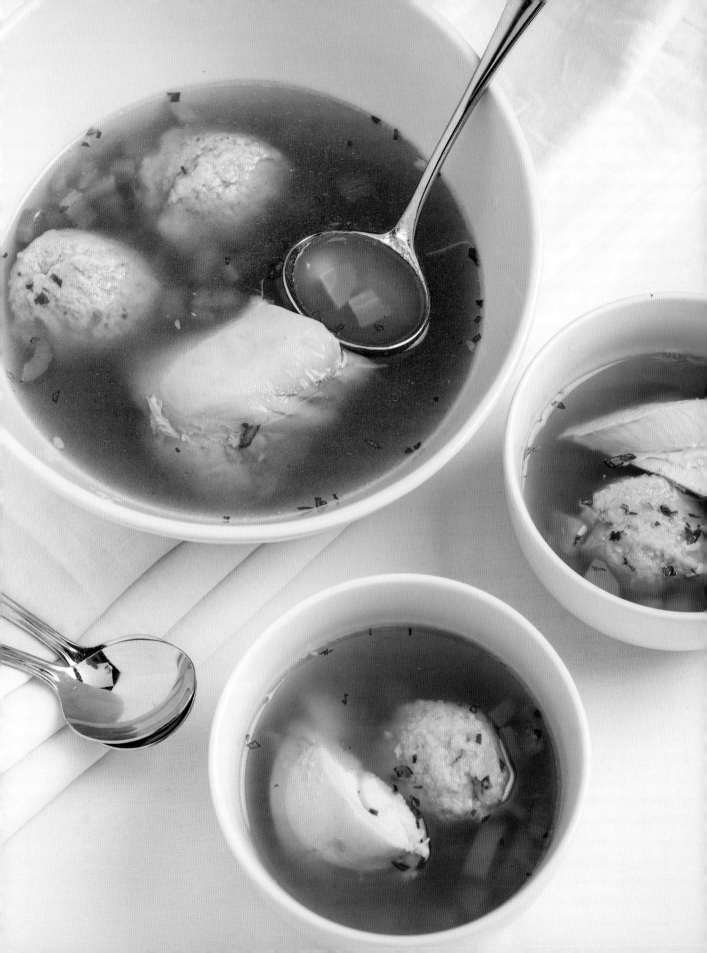

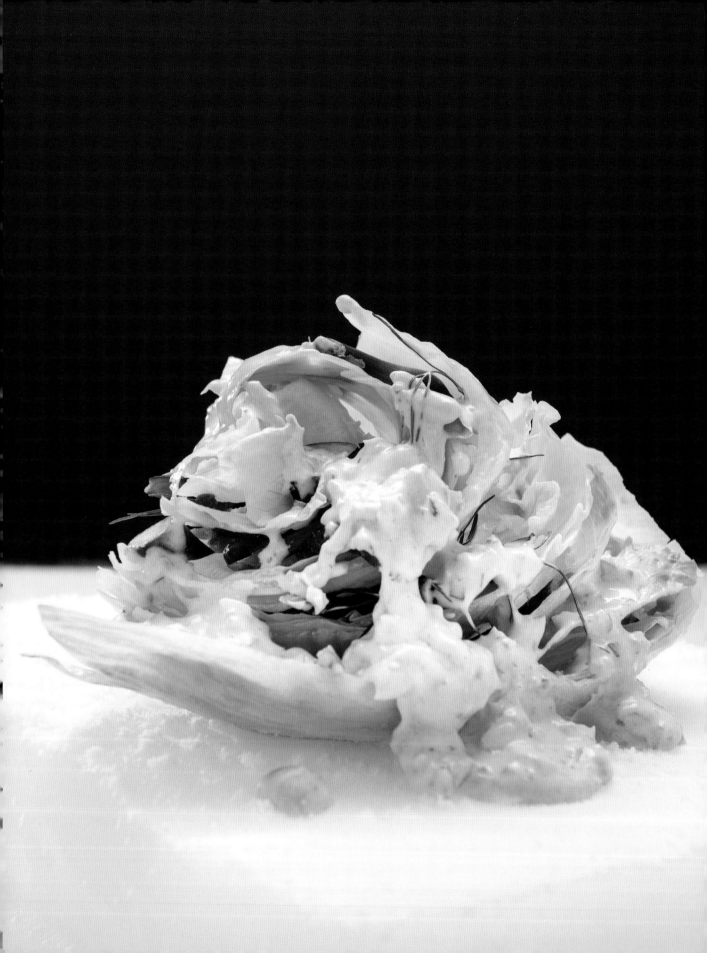

Wedge Salad with House Dressing

YIELD: 4 APPETIZER SERVINGS

Go big or go home. That was always Eli's philosophy, and it applied to everything Eli's The Place For Steak served. In order for the salad to be the same scale as a steak, Eli's vision was to create a big wedge of crisp, cold iceberg lettuce topped with a generous dollop of his house dressing—there was nothing better. Remember when Barbra Streisand's character in The Mirror Has Two Faces *orders a salad with "more dressing and a side of extra dressing"? That's how our daughter Elana likes it, too.*

1 head iceberg lettuce, washed and crisped and cut into four equal wedges

4 strips cooked smoked bacon, crumbled

1 recipe The Place For Steak House Dressing (recipe on p. 62)

1 handful fennel fronds, for garnish

1. Place the four lettuce wedges, flat side down, on chilled shallow dishes or plates. Either scatter the bacon crumbles over the lettuce wedges or stuff them into the wedges.

2. Pour Eli's House Dressing on top of the lettuce wedges. Garnish with the fennel fronds and serve immediately.

NOTE: If any of the dressing is left over, you can add 2 teaspoons of vinegar to it and store it covered in the refrigerator for up to 5 days. This classic mid-century salad dressing will jazz up even the palest of iceberg lettuces and is a perfect mayonnaise substitute on any salad or sandwich.

Eli's The Place For Steak House Dressing

YIELD: 6 SERVINGS

3 large hard-boiled egg whites, room temperature, finely chopped

2½ cups mayonnaise

1 large green bell pepper

1 large red bell pepper

1 medium onion, chopped

½ cup red chili sauce, drained

½ cup finely chopped fresh Italian parsley

½ cup sweet pickle relish, drained

1. In a medium mixing bowl, combine the egg whites and mayonnaise.

2. In the bowl of a food processor fitted with the "S" blade, combine the green and red bell peppers. Pulse the mixture, pausing to scrape down the sides of the bowl, until the peppers are finely grated and semi-liquid. Spread the processed peppers on a bed of paper towels and blot them dry. Transfer the dried peppers to the egg white–mayonnaise mixture and stir to combine.

3. Press the red chili sauce through a medium wire strainer; doing so will yield approximately 2 tablespoons of solid material still clinging to the strainer. Scrape the solid material into the bowl containing the egg white–mayonnaise mixture. Repeat the same process with the pickle relish. Stir until thoroughly combined.

4. Place the mixing bowl in the refrigerator and chill for 2 to 3 hours before serving.

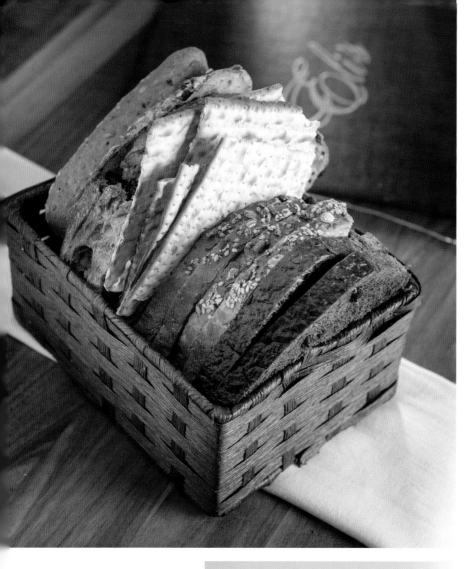

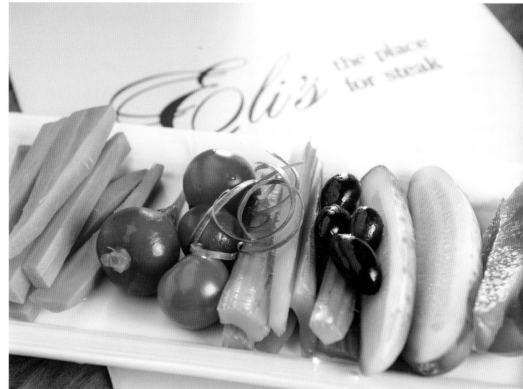

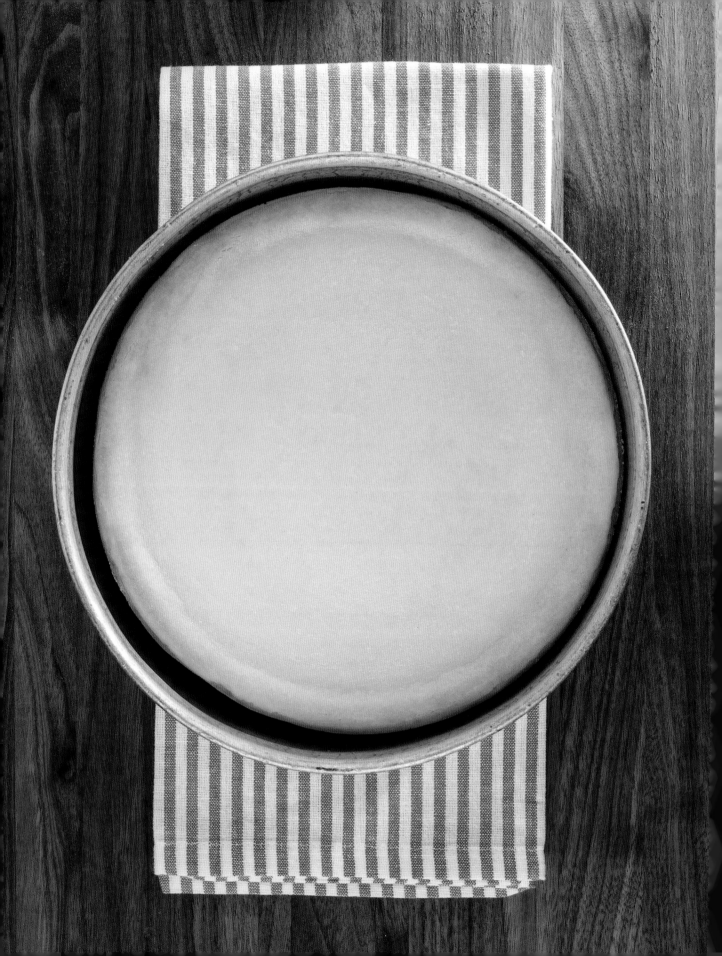

ELI'S DELICIOUS DESSERTS

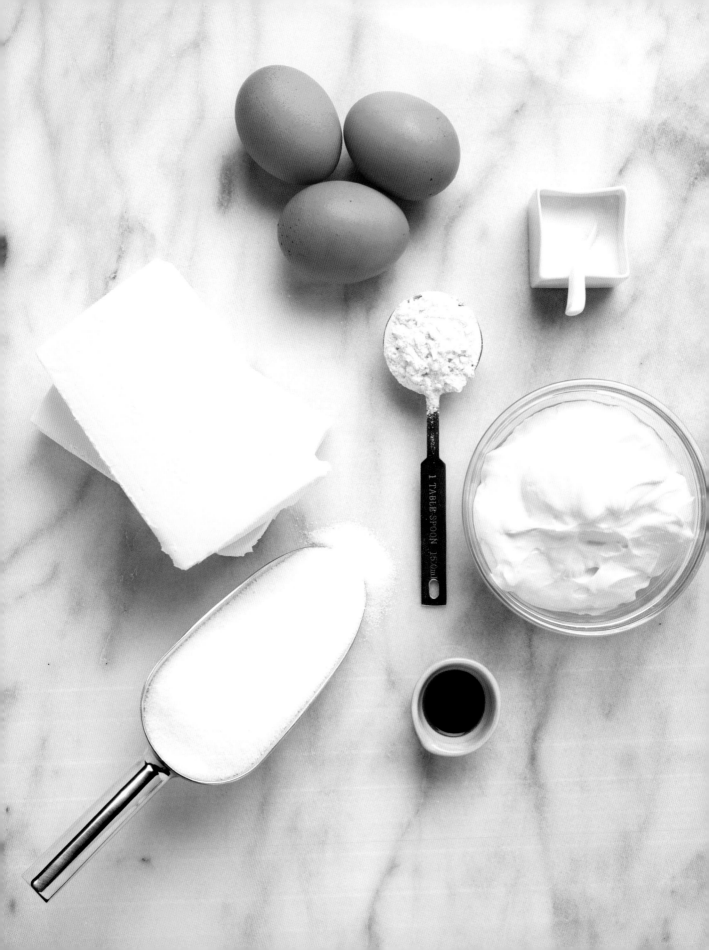

Pure, Plain, and Simple: The One that Started It All

"Eli dispelled everything we knew about cheesecake." —Jolene Worthington

PERFECTING THE CHEESECAKE

When Jolene Worthington first arrived at The Eli's Cheesecake Company, Eli himself presented her with a cheesecake and charged her with the task of making every cheesecake perfect on a much larger scale and also adding more varieties to the lineup. Jolene, a superb, classically trained pastry chef, was game for the challenge; she approached the project in a very scientific manner. After all, baking is a science. When she experienced that first cheesecake, she was surprised at how beautiful it was, with its golden-brown caramelized top. "It had structure, and yet, it was a quivering custard inside," said Jolene. In fact, she found that the cheesecake demonstrated so much inner strength that it could survive being tossed like a Frisbee on its journey from oven to cooling rack. Jolene realized then and there that although Eli had broken all the rules when it came to baking this new breed of cheesecake—no water bath, bake hot and fast—he had managed to unlock the secret of how to soufflé a rich, dense custard into a perfect cheesecake. That's Chicago-style cheesecake.

Jolene created a standard of identity for The Eli's Cheesecake Company by figuring out how to replicate Eli's idea of a perfect cheesecake every time—what ingredients worked best, what temperatures achieved the signature golden color and caramelized top, and what baking times provided the best lift and structure.

The first few years of her work were characterized by trial and error. As Jolene switched from fifty-cake batches to batches of a few hundred at a time, new issues occasionally arose:

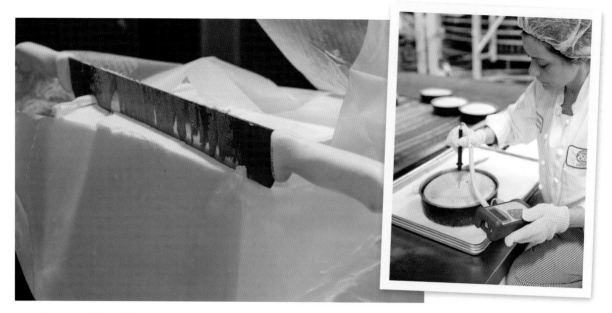

A 50-pound block of Eli's custom cream cheese.

Diana takes the internal temperature of a cheesecake.

some of the cakes cracked, collapsed, or exhibited other imperfections. To combat these variations, Jolene, Diana, and the rest of the cheesecake "whisperers" set out on a mission to figure out why, despite the fact that they were performing every step—tempering the ingredients, maintaining the same mixing times, baking times, and temperatures—in the same way each time, these problems kept occurring.

They discovered that not all ingredients are created equal. Different brands of cream cheese, sugar, sour cream, and even eggs all performed differently in the various batters. And even within the same brands, they occasionally found inconsistencies. The answer: Ordering ingredients in quantities large enough that the suppliers were willing to customize them in order to ensure consistency on all fronts. But at home, you don't have to worry about baking hundreds of identical cakes at a time. Store-bought ingredients may vary, but rest assured that we have carefully tested these recipes in home kitchens, one cheesecake at a time, over the course of several months using ingredients from a variety of brands. These recipes are tried and true, and take ingredient variances into consideration.

Anyone reading this cookbook is the lucky beneficiary of more than 35 years of cheesecake know-how. Our scientific testing of ingredients and techniques will help you solve any cheesecake problems that may arise. This cookbook is divided into sections for Batters, Crusts, and Finishing Touches, and you'll find some of our favorite combinations in Putting It

All Together. This system offers so much flexibility and opportunity for creativity that if you combined one option from each section, you could bake 2,860 different cheesecakes! *The Eli's Cheesecake Cookbook* doesn't just give you delicious recipes; it empowers you, the home cook, with the knowledge and science behind baking the perfect cheesecake.

WHAT IS A CHICAGO-STYLE ELI'S ORIGINAL PLAIN?

Our cheesecake is simple—and that's why it's so good. We start with the cornerstone custard ingredients: sugar, eggs, and vanilla. Our recipe involves using a heavy mixer paddle to blend sugar, flour, and salt into thick slabs of cream cheese until the mixture becomes emulsified, or embedded with small air pockets. The small quantity of flour is there to improve the cheesecake's mouth feel, helping transfer all those creamy fats to the tongue. Later on, we slowly mix in whole eggs and egg yolks. The mixture doubles in volume and becomes thick, yet vulnerable, like a soufflé. Last, we fold in cultured sour cream; its high fat content lends the cheesecake its luxurious taste.

The Ingredients

CULTURED CREAM CHEESE has been the structural backbone of American cheesecakes since Kraft first began to produce it in 1912. By the 1930s, when cheesecake recipes began appearing in cookbooks, cultured cream cheese became a convenient replacement for more traditional cheese. European immigrants traditionally churned separated, semi-solid, soured cream to make simple soft pot cheeses like cottage cheese, quark, and ricotta, as well as thick yogurts. Cultured cream cheese has a unique sweet and tangy flavor that comes from lactic acid, a by-product of the bacteria *Lactococcus*. This beneficial bacterium is necessary to produce the fermentation required to make crème fraîche, yogurt, and cheese.

The Eli's Cheesecake Company only uses cultured fresh cream cheese and cultured sour cream. Adding fillers, stabilizers, or artificial ingredients ruins the simple custard taste and can lead to a dry and flavorless cake. Whether you bake it or set it with gelatin, cheesecake derives its body; its unique sweet, tangy flavor; and its perfect mouth feel from the 33 percent milk fat of the cream and milk in the cream cheese. The cultures added to the milk and cream ferment the mixture, generating the naturally occurring metabolic lactic acids. The

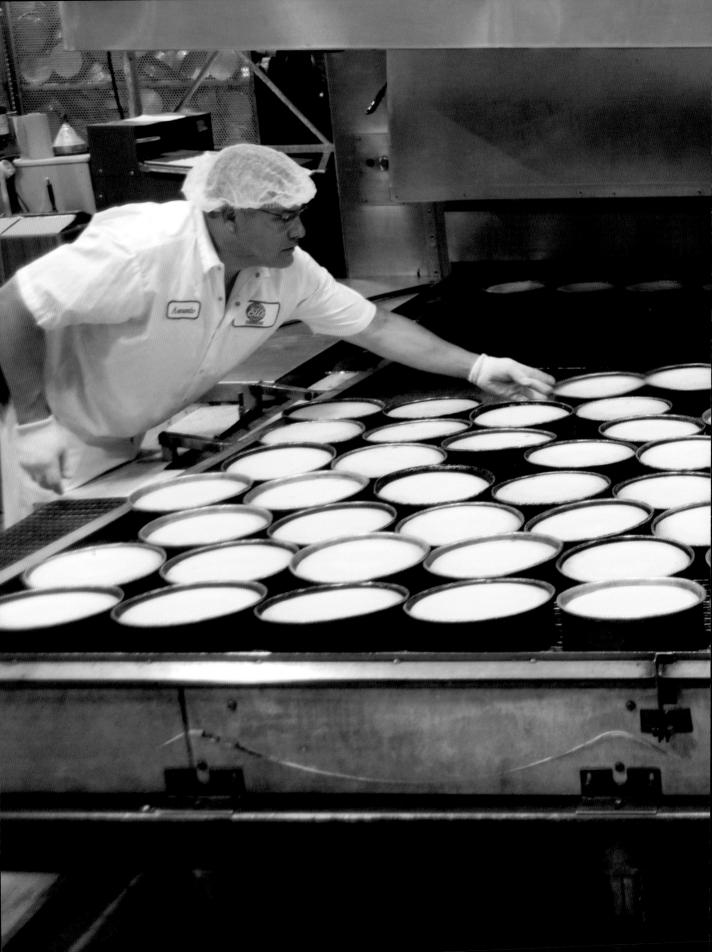

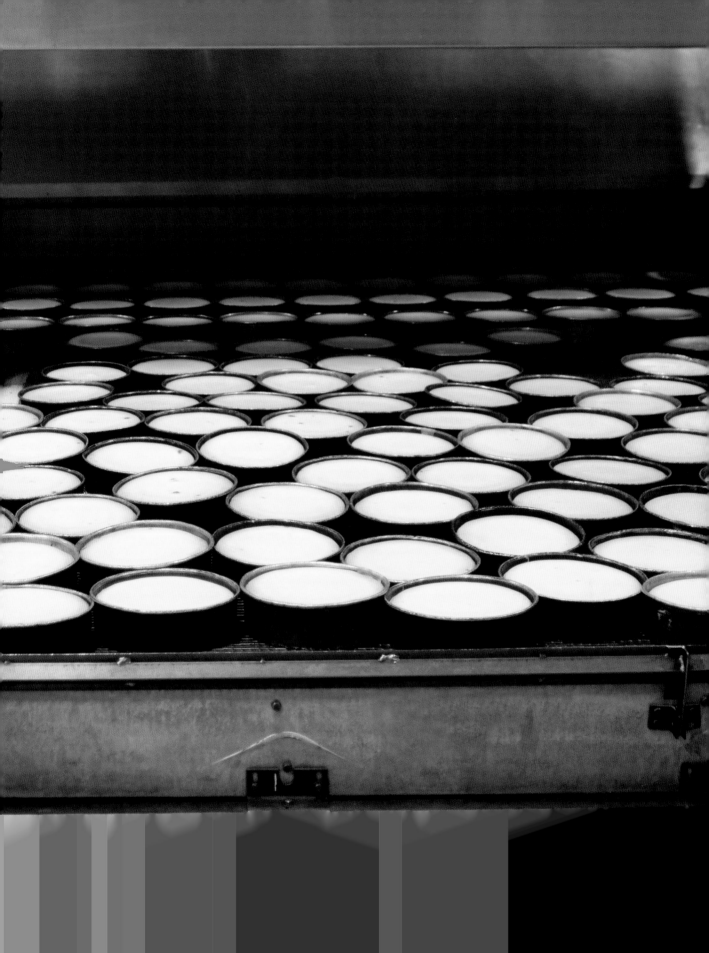

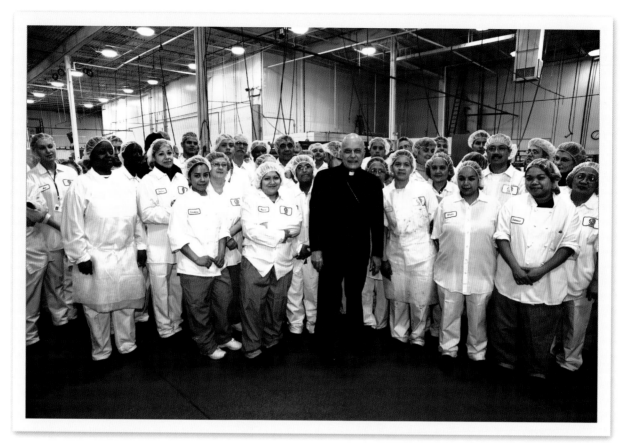

The late Francis Cardinal George visiting Eli's bakery production floor. Marc's first assistant, Rita Tierny, arranged for Eli's to send cheesecakes to Rome for the Cardinal's induction. Eli's is very near where the Cardinal grew up and attended St. Pascal's Parish.

acids quickly flourish and give body and sweetness to the culture. We only use real cream cheese—never "cream cheese blends" that aren't all dairy. Because different brands of cream cheese have their own characteristic flavors, you should try several in order to select the one that tastes best to you. Pick one with a clean, sweet cheese flavor.

SOUR CREAM is also cultured. Just as with the cream cheese, the process produces a sweet taste that rounds out the natural lactic acid flavor notes in the batter. Diana Moles, vice president of research and development at The Eli's Cheesecake Company, remarked, "We are so picky about our ingredients that we went to the dairy supplier and tested the sour cream every hour for 18 hours to achieve the perfect flavor and pH for our cheesecakes." We don't recommend acidified, noncultured, or "light" sour creams for any of our recipes, but crème fraîche is a tangy cousin to cultured sour cream that can replace the sour cream in our recipes. Sour cream will lighten the density of the cheesecake's body as it whips faster and denser than whipped cream.

SUGAR adds sweetness and aids in the browning process. The sugar also allows these high-fat cheesecakes to be frozen and thawed without suffering any structural damage, as it helps produce small ice crystals like those found in ice cream.

EGGS govern the lightness, density, and structure of a cheesecake more than any other ingredient. A whole range of cheesecake textures can be achieved simply by manipulating the quantity of eggs in the batter. The egg's yolk and white are both key ingredients that help emulsify, stabilize, and add body and flavor to a wide variety of desserts. With each bite of cheesecake you can feel the richness the yolks add to the batter and see the delicate amber color it adds to the finished dessert. The egg white, the other half of the miracle ingredient, adds protein and when whipped makes meringue to create a delicate texture.

FLOUR does not play an important structural role in cheesecake formulation. It is responsible for helping deliver flavorful caramelization of the crust and the desirable mouth feel one looks for in cheesecake.

VANILLA is a crucial flavor component of all Eli's cheesecakes. We use only pure Madagascar Bourbon vanilla extract and vanilla beans from Nielsen-Massey Vanilla, a Certified Fair Trade company headquartered in Waukegan, Illinois. There, the very finest, handpicked vanilla beans undergo an exclusive cold extraction process that creates one of the finest vanilla extracts in the world. Like Eli's, Nielsen-Massey is a family-owned business committed to quality and high standards.

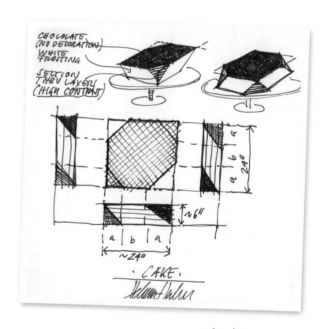

After doing a project with the world-renowned architect Helmut Jahn to benefit the Chicago Children's Museum, Marc and Maureen asked him to sketch the perfect cheesecake.

DEMYSTIFYING THE CHEESECAKE

TEMPERING AND MIXING: One of the most critical secrets at Eli's involves tempering all the dairy ingredients used in our cakes' batters. The cream cheese, eggs, and sour cream—so essential to the perfect Eli's cheesecake—must reach room temperature prior to mixing. Cold cream cheese is very hard and difficult to aerate during the mixing process. All the little air cells needed to hold the rich fats together aren't present if the cream cheese doesn't have an opportunity to warm and soften.

The mixing process causes the fats to cream together, which is known as emulsification. In the case of a cheesecake, the emulsification process combines the cream cheese, eggs, and sour cream with the sugar, flour, and vanilla. Our cheesecake batters are mixed slowly and for a long period of time, which causes a chemical exchange of molecules that adds air to the batter. In a cheesecake, this air leavens the batter and enhances its tenderness and flavor.

Another critical step is using an upright stand mixer or hand mixer instead of a food processor to emulsify the batter. It takes 15 minutes to properly mix an Eli's cheesecake, adding one ingredient at a time and scraping down the bowl after adding each ingredient. The high-speed blades of food processors can shear the proteins in the batter, which ultimately may collapse the cake.

If after the mixing process, you find that your batter is extremely runny instead of fluffy and thick, your dairy ingredients may have been too cold. You also may have overmixed the batter, which collapses the emulsification process and may cause the baked cake to crack or to fail to soufflé.

THE PAN: Our baking pans have flat, removable bottoms for easy removal of the cakes. They're metal, which is essential for good heat transfer. Before the crusts are firmly packed in and the batters are poured, the pans are lightly greased and floured.

THE METHOD: A key technique to baking an Eli's cheesecake is to start at a very high temperature and then reduce the temperature as the baking process continues. Many cheesecake recipes require a water bath (also known as a *bain-marie*), but ours do not. At Eli's, we find that a very hot, dry oven helps evaporate the cheesecake's excess moisture, allowing the cake's surface to become lightly browned and mottled, like a well-caramelized custard. The

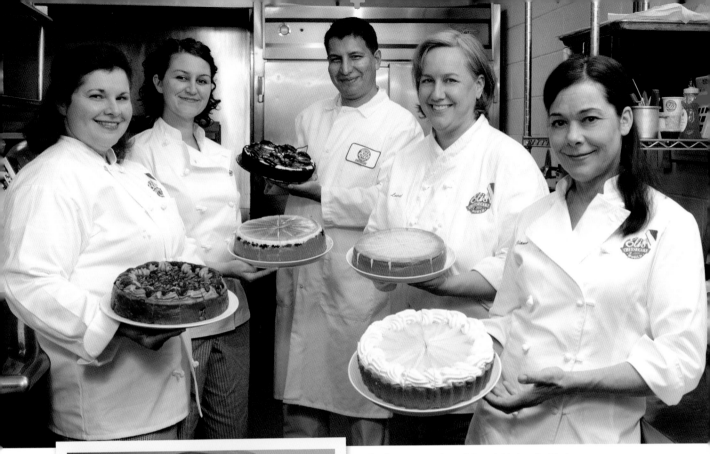

Eli's dream team, shown left to right: Juanita Chajon,
Tara Lane, Aurelio Ayala, Laurel Boger, and Diana Moles.
PHOTO BY VITO PALMISANO.

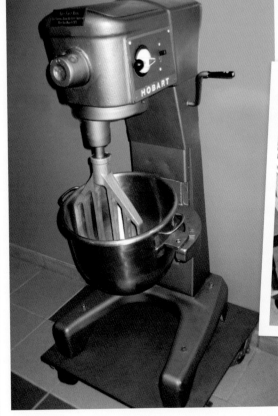

Eli's first mixer, 1980.   Decorators swirl raspberry coulis
into cheesecake batter.

high heat caramelizes the top, which traps steam underneath and actually cooks the cake.

Another benefit of baking at a high temperature: Rapidly vaporizing the moisture in the batter helps inflate its air pockets, just like a soufflé. Sure enough, Eli's cheesecakes rise out of the pan like soufflés. Once an Eli's cheesecake comes out of the oven and rests, it continues to bake and release more steam until it slightly deflates into a firm, custard center.

How do we know when our cheesecakes are done? Here's another secret: Eli's expert bakers always remove the cheesecakes from the oven while they're still very soft, jiggle a bit in the center, and appear not quite yet done. We know that the cake's internal temperature will continue to rise another 5 to 10 degrees after it comes out of the oven, and thus it will continue to cook.

Transferring from Oven, Cooling, and Cutting:
We don't disturb a cheesecake fresh out of the oven until its proteins have had a chance to coagulate and become firm, which takes at least 45 minutes to an hour. Too much handling can crack the cake's surface. After a cheesecake sits for an hour at room temperature, we immediately release it from the sides of the pan and leave it sitting on the pan's metal bottom. At that point, you can refrigerate your cheesecake overnight or even wrap it carefully and freeze it for 3 to 6 months before enjoying it.

Yet another secret: Everyone knows that cheesecakes are difficult to cut. At Eli's, we freeze cheesecakes before we cut them, which leaves every slice with smooth, even sides.

ELI'S TRADE SECRET

DON'T FORGET THE SIX CRITICAL STEPS:

1. Make sure your eggs, cream cheese, and sour cream are warmed to room temperature.

2. During the mixing process, scrape the sides and bottom of the bowl after you add each ingredient.

3. Always mix the sugar and flour together before adding it to the cream cheese mixture.

4. You may be used to using just butter or cooking spray to coat your pan. At Eli's, our trade secret is blending flour and vegetable oil to ensure an easy pan release. The addition of flour also creates a caramelization and golden color on the sides of your cheesecake. Simply whisk three tablespoons vegetable oil to one tablespoon all-purpose flour and generously brush the sides of the pan with a pastry brush or a paper towel.

5. Start baking at a very high temperature and then reduce the temperature as the baking process continues. Eli's expert bakers always remove cheesecakes while they're still very soft, jiggle a bit in the center, and appear not quite yet done.

6. Allow the cheesecake to sit undisturbed in its pan for about an hour after it comes out of the oven.

BATTERS

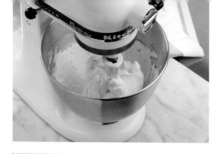

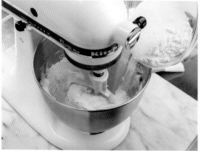

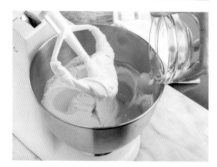

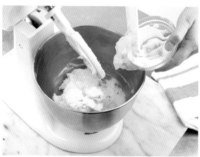

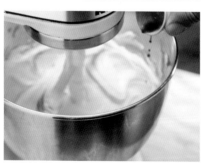

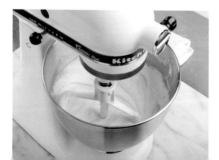

Original Plain Cheesecake

YIELD: 1 (9-INCH) SPRINGFORM CHEESECAKE / 12 SERVINGS

4 (8-ounce) packages cream cheese, room temperature

1 cup granulated sugar

¼ cup cake flour

¼ teaspoon salt

2 large whole eggs, room temperature

1 large egg yolk, room temperature

¾ cup sour cream, room temperature

1 teaspoon vanilla extract

1. In the bowl of a stand mixer fitted with the paddle attachment, beat the cream cheese on medium speed for 2 to 3 minutes, until it is light and fluffy. Scrape down the sides and bottom of the stand mixer bowl to prevent lumps from forming.

2. In a separate medium mixing bowl, combine the sugar, cake flour, and salt. Stir until well combined.

3. Add the contents of the medium mixing bowl to the bowl of the stand mixer and beat on medium speed for 1 minute. Scrape down the sides and bottom of the stand mixer bowl and continue beating on medium speed for 1 to 2 minutes, until the mixture is smooth and creamy.

4. Reduce the mixer speed to low. Slowly add first the whole eggs and then the egg yolk to the bowl, one at a time. After adding each, scrape down the sides and bottom of the bowl. Continue beating on low speed for 1 to 2 minutes, until the mixture is fully incorporated.

5. Add the sour cream and the vanilla to the bowl of the stand mixer and beat on low speed for 1 minute, until the mixture is smooth. The mixture should be well blended, but not overbeaten.

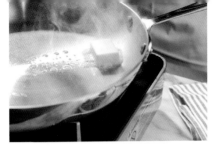

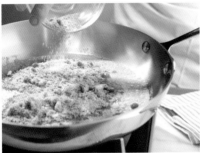

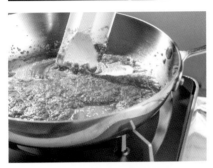

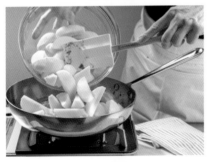

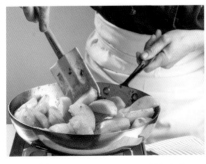

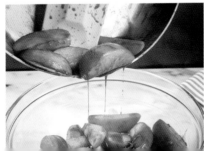

Baked Apple

YIELD: 1 (9-INCH) SPRINGFORM CHEESECAKE / 12 SERVINGS

APPLES:

2 tablespoons unsalted butter

6 baking (Ida Red or Northern Spy) apples, peeled, cored, and cut into 1-inch-thick wedges

¼ cup granulated sugar

¼ cup light brown sugar

1 teaspoon ground cinnamon

CHEESECAKE:

4 (8-ounce) packages cream cheese, room temperature

1 cup granulated sugar

¼ cup cake flour

¼ teaspoon salt

2 large whole eggs, room temperature

1 large egg yolk, room temperature

¾ cup sour cream, room temperature

1 teaspoon vanilla extract

1. *Prepare the apples:* Place a large saucepan over medium heat. Add the butter.

2. In a large mixing bowl, combine the sugars and the cinnamon and stir until well combined. Once the butter in the saucepan has melted, add the sugar mixture to the saucepan and cook for 5 minutes, until the sugar begins to caramelize. Place the apple wedges in the caramelized mixture and sauté for 5 minutes, until the apples are slightly firm to the touch, but not overcooked. (Keep in mind, the apples will be baked a second time.) Remove from the heat and set aside.

3. *Prepare the cheesecake:* In the bowl of a stand mixer fitted with the paddle attachment, beat the cream cheese on medium speed for 2 to 3 minutes, until it is light and fluffy. Scrape down the sides and bottom of the stand mixer bowl to prevent lumps from forming.

RECIPE CONTINUES ON PAGE 80

4. In a separate medium mixing bowl, combine the sugar, cake flour, and salt. Stir until well combined.

5. Add the contents of the medium mixing bowl to the bowl of the stand mixer and beat on medium speed for 1 minute. Scrape down the sides and bottom of the stand mixer bowl and continue beating on medium speed for 2 to 3 minutes, until the mixture is smooth and creamy.

6. Reduce the mixer speed to low. Slowly add first the whole eggs and then the egg yolk to the bowl, one at a time. After adding each, scrape down the sides and bottom of the bowl. Continue beating on low speed for 1 to 2 minutes, until the mixture is fully incorporated.

7. Add the sour cream and the vanilla to the bowl of the stand mixer and beat on low speed for 1 minute, until the mixture is smooth. The mixture should be well blended, but not overbeaten.

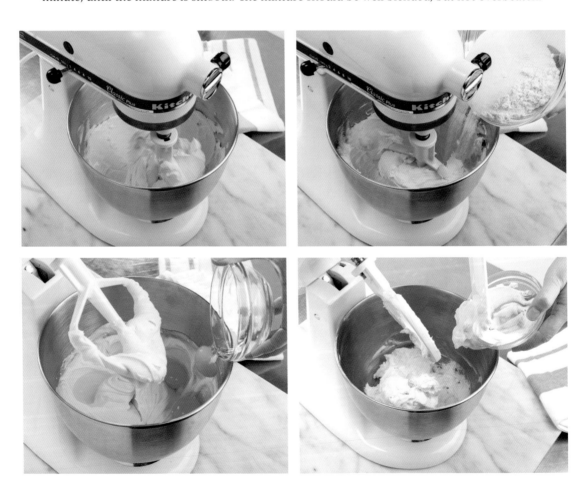

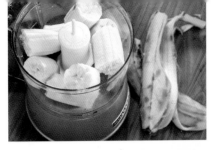

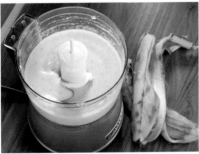

Banana

YIELD: 2 (6-INCH) SPRINGFORM CHEESECAKES / 12 SERVINGS

2 (8-ounce) packages cream cheese, room temperature

¾ cup light brown sugar

2 tablespoons cake flour

2 large whole eggs, room temperature

2 large ripe bananas, puréed (should yield 1 cup)

½ teaspoon vanilla extract

¼ cup sour cream, room temperature

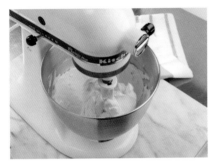

1. In the bowl of a stand mixer fitted with the paddle attachment, beat the cream cheese on medium speed for 2 to 3 minutes, until it is light and fluffy. Scrape down the sides and bottom of the stand mixer bowl to prevent lumps from forming.

2. In a separate small mixing bowl, combine the sugar and cake flour. Stir until well combined.

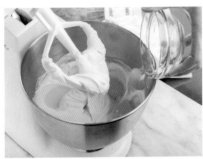

3. Add the contents of the small mixing bowl to the bowl of the stand mixer and beat on medium speed for 1 minute. Scrape down the sides and bottom of the stand mixer bowl and continue beating on medium speed for 2 to 3 minutes, until the mixture is smooth and creamy.

4. Reduce the mixer speed to low. Slowly add the eggs to the bowl, one at a time. After adding each, scrape down the sides and bottom of the bowl. Continue beating on low speed for 1 to 2 minutes, until the mixture is fully incorporated.

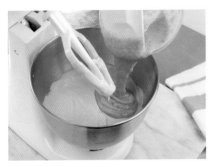

5. Add the puréed bananas and the vanilla to the bowl of the stand mixer and beat on low speed for 1 minute, until the mixture is smooth.

6. Add the sour cream to the bowl of the stand mixer and beat on low speed for 1 minute, until the sour cream is just incorporated. The mixture should be well blended, but not overbeaten.

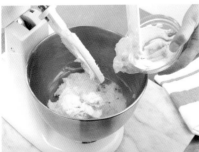

Belgian Chocolate

YIELD: 1 (14-INCH × 4.5-INCH × 1-INCH) RECTANGULAR TART / 8 SERVINGS

1 (8-ounce) package cream cheese, room temperature

⅓ cup granulated sugar

1 tablespoon cocoa powder

2 large whole eggs, room temperature

½ teaspoon vanilla extract

8 ounces Belgian Chocolate Ganache (recipe follows)

1. In the bowl of a stand mixer fitted with the paddle attachment, beat the cream cheese on medium speed for 2 to 3 minutes, until it is light and fluffy. Scrape down the sides and bottom of the stand mixer bowl to prevent lumps from forming.

2. In a separate small mixing bowl, combine the sugar and cocoa powder. Stir until well combined.

3. Add the contents of the small mixing bowl to the bowl of the stand mixer and beat on medium speed for 1 minute. Scrape down the sides and bottom of the stand mixer bowl and continue beating on medium speed for 2 to 3 minutes, until the mixture is smooth and creamy.

4. Reduce the mixer speed to low. Slowly add the eggs to the bowl, one at a time. After adding each, scrape down the sides and bottom of the bowl. Continue beating on low speed for 1 to 2 minutes, until the mixture is fully incorporated.

5. Add the vanilla and the Belgian Chocolate Ganache to the bowl of the stand mixer and beat on low speed for 1 to 2 minutes, until the mixture is just combined. Scrape down the sides of the bowl. The mixture should be well blended, but not overbeaten.

VARIATIONS

Spiced Belgian Chocolate Cheesecake: Add 1 teaspoon of ground cinnamon to the small mixing bowl in Step 2.

Belgian Chocolate and Mint Cheesecake: After the batter is completely mixed, gently fold 5 ounces of miniature mint chocolate chips into it using a spatula, making sure the chips are well dispersed.

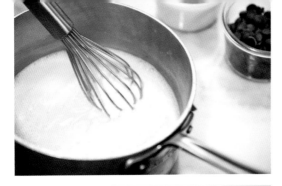

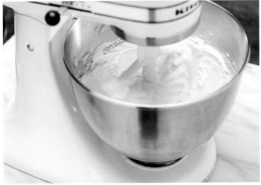

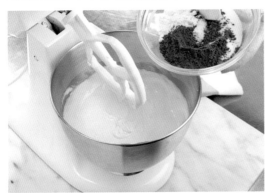

Belgian Chocolate Ganache

YIELD: 8 OUNCES

5 ounces Belgian bittersweet chocolate

⅓ cup heavy cream

1. Chop the chocolate into small pieces. Place the chocolate in a medium heatproof mixing bowl.

2. Place the heavy cream in a small saucepan over medium heat. Cook for 3 to 4 minutes, until a skin begins to form on the cream. Remove from the heat.

3. Transfer the heated cream to the medium mixing bowl containing the chocolate. Set aside for 1 minute to allow the chocolate to begin to melt.

4. Whisk the mixture vigorously, until it is smooth and all the chocolate has melted. Cover with plastic wrap and set aside.

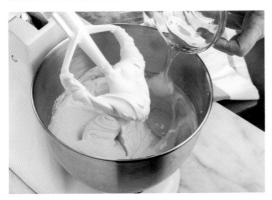

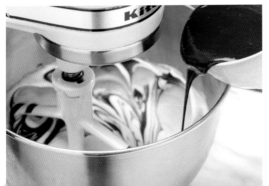

Chocolate Chip

YIELD: 1 (9-INCH) SPRINGFORM CHEESECAKE / 12 SERVINGS

4 (8-ounce) packages cream cheese, room temperature

1 cup granulated sugar

¼ cup cake flour

¼ teaspoon salt

2 large whole eggs, room temperature

1 large egg yolk, room temperature

¾ cup sour cream, room temperature

½ teaspoon vanilla extract

1½ cups + 1 tablespoon miniature bittersweet chocolate chips

1. In the bowl of a stand mixer fitted with the paddle attachment, beat the cream cheese on medium speed for 2 to 3 minutes, until it is light and fluffy. Scrape down the sides and bottom of the stand mixer bowl to prevent lumps from forming.

2. In a separate medium mixing bowl, combine the sugar, cake flour, and salt. Stir until well combined.

3. Add the contents of the medium mixing bowl to the bowl of the stand mixer and beat on medium speed for 1 minute. Scrape down the sides and bottom of the stand mixer bowl and continue beating on medium speed for 2 to 3 minutes, until the mixture is smooth and creamy.

4. Reduce the mixer speed to low. Slowly add first the whole eggs and then the egg yolk to the bowl, one at a time. After adding each, scrape down the sides and bottom of the bowl. Continue beating on low speed for 1 to 2 minutes, until the mixture is fully incorporated.

5. Add the sour cream and the vanilla to the bowl of the stand mixer and beat on low speed for 1 minute, until the mixture is smooth. The mixture should be well blended, but not overbeaten.

6. Gently fold the 1½ cups chocolate chips into the batter, until evenly dispersed. Reserve the 1 tablespoon chocolate chips to evenly sprinkle over the top of the batter once it is placed in the pan.

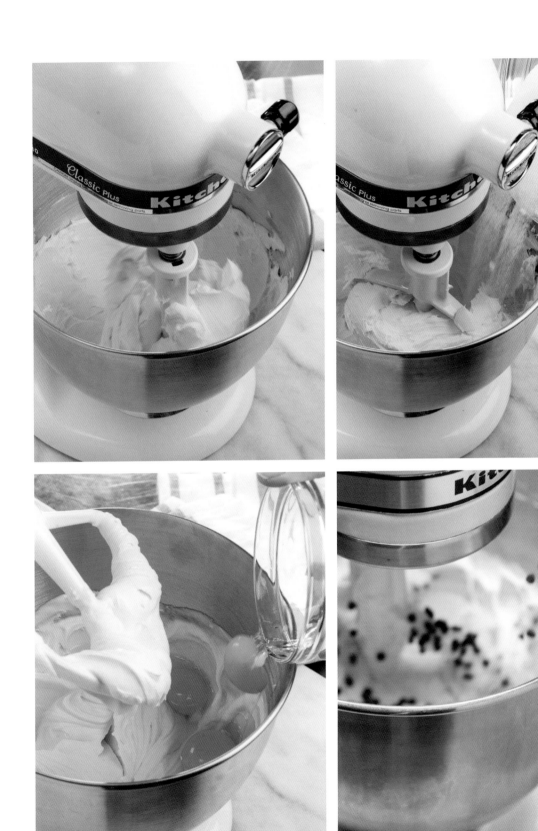

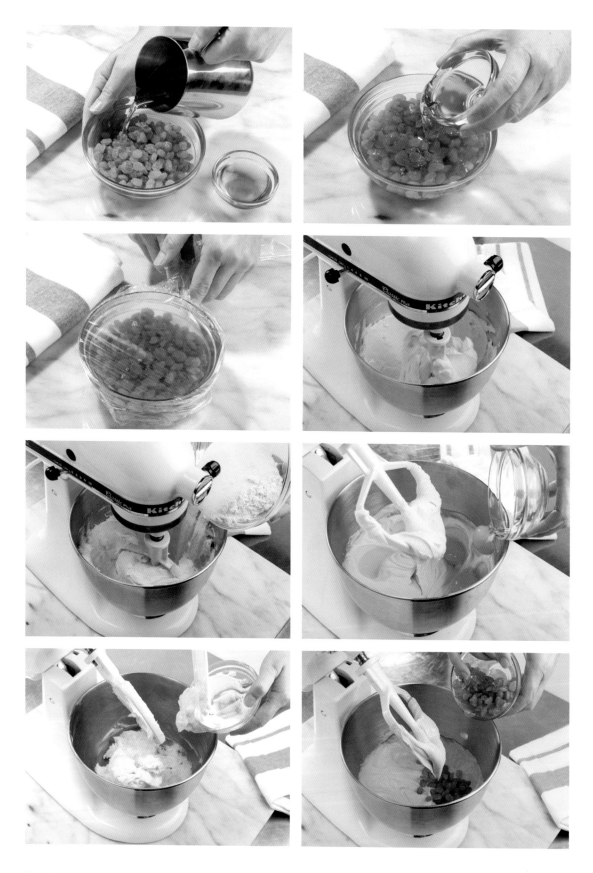

Cinnamon Rum Raisin

YIELD: 1 (9-INCH) SPRINGFORM CHEESECAKE OR 2 (6-INCH) SPRINGFORM CHEESECAKES / 12 SERVINGS

PLUMPED RAISINS:

1 cup golden raisins

1 cup boiling water

¼ cup dark rum

2 tablespoons unsalted butter

CHEESECAKE:

4 (8-ounce) packages cream cheese, room temperature

1 cup granulated sugar

¼ cup cake flour

½ teaspoon ground cinnamon

¼ teaspoon salt

2 large whole eggs, room temperature

1 large egg yolk, room temperature

¾ cup sour cream, room temperature

1 teaspoon vanilla extract

1. In a medium heatproof glass bowl, combine the raisins, water, and rum. Cover the bowl with plastic wrap and set aside to steep for at least 5 minutes, until the raisins have plumped.

2. In the bowl of a stand mixer fitted with the paddle attachment, beat the cream cheese on medium speed for 2 to 3 minutes, until it is light and fluffy. Scrape down the sides and bottom of the stand mixer bowl to prevent lumps from forming.

3. In a separate medium mixing bowl, combine the sugar, cake flour, cinnamon, and salt. Stir until well combined.

4. Add the contents of the medium mixing bowl to the bowl of the stand mixer and beat on medium speed for 1 minute. Scrape down the sides and bottom of the stand mixer bowl and continue beating on medium speed for 2 to 3 minutes, until the mixture is smooth and creamy.

5. Reduce the mixer speed to low. Slowly add first the whole eggs and then the egg yolk to the bowl, one at a time. After adding each, scrape down the sides and bottom of the bowl. Continue beating on low speed for 1 to 2 minutes, until the mixture is fully incorporated.

6. Add the sour cream and the vanilla to the bowl of the stand mixer and beat on low speed for 1 minute, until the mixture is smooth. The mixture should be well blended, but not overbeaten.

7. Drain the raisins and gently fold them into the batter, until evenly dispersed.

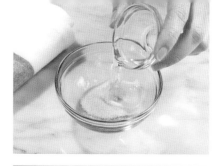

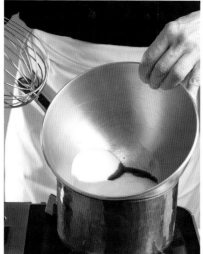

Crème Fraîche No-Bake

YIELD: 8 (4-OUNCE) SERVINGS

1 teaspoon unflavored gelatin powder

2 teaspoons cold water

2 cups water

2/3 cup granulated sugar, divided

2 large egg yolks, room temperature

2 (8-ounce) packages cream cheese, room temperature

3/4 cup crème fraîche

1 cup heavy cream

1 teaspoon vanilla extract

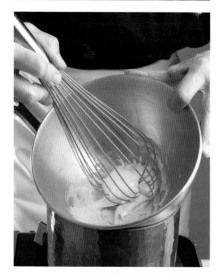

1. In a small mixing bowl, stir together the gelatin powder and the cold water. Set aside to bloom.

2. *Make a sabayon:* Place the 2 cups of water in a saucepan over medium–high heat and bring to a boil. Place a medium heatproof bowl on top of the boiling water and add ⅓ cup of the sugar and the egg yolks to the bowl. Whisk vigorously until fluffy ribbons form in the mixture and its temperature reaches 150°F. Remove from the heat and whisk in the bloomed gelatin until the mixture is fully combined. Set aside.

3. In the bowl of a stand mixer fitted with the paddle attachment, beat the cream cheese on medium speed for 2 to 3 minutes, until it is smooth and free of lumps.

4. Resume mixing at medium speed. One at a time, add the remaining ⅓ cup of the sugar, the crème fraîche, and the heavy cream to the bowl of the stand mixer and beat on medium speed for 1 to 2 minutes, until the mixture is smooth and creamy. Scrape down the sides and bottom of the stand mixer bowl and add the vanilla. Using a wooden spoon or silicone spatula, stir until fully combined.

5. Fold the cream cheese mixture into the sabayon. Pour immediately into serving containers to set.

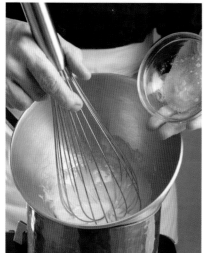

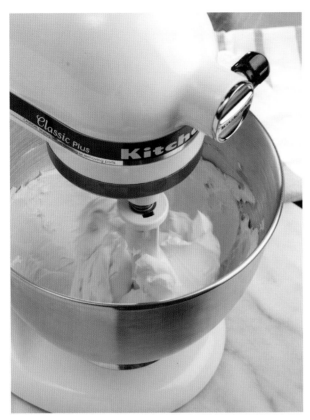

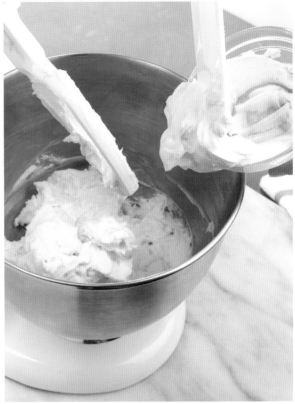

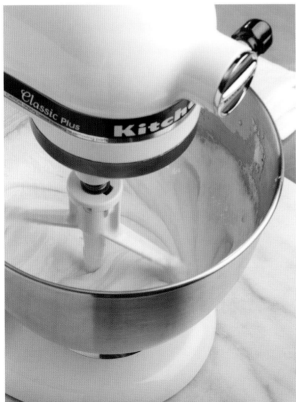

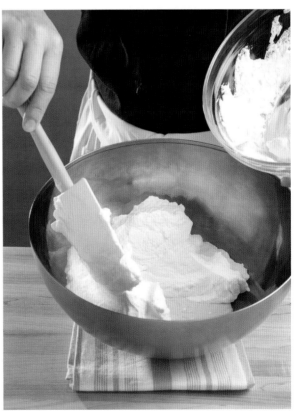

Eggnog

3 (8-ounce) packages cream cheese, room temperature

1 cup granulated sugar

¼ cup cake flour

1 teaspoon ground nutmeg

4 large egg yolks, room temperature

1 cup eggnog, divided, room temperature

½ teaspoon vanilla extract

2 tablespoons dark rum (optional)

1. In the bowl of a stand mixer fitted with the paddle attachment, beat the cream cheese on medium speed for 2 to 3 minutes, until it is light and fluffy. Scrape down the sides and bottom of the stand mixer bowl to prevent lumps from forming.

2. In a separate medium mixing bowl, combine the sugar, cake flour, and nutmeg. Stir until well combined.

3. Add the contents of the medium mixing bowl to the bowl of the stand mixer and beat on medium speed for 1 minute. Scrape down the sides and bottom of the stand mixer bowl and continue beating on medium speed for 2 to 3 minutes, until the mixture is smooth and creamy.

4. Reduce the mixer speed to low. Slowly add the egg yolks to the bowl, one at a time. After adding each yolk, scrape down the sides and bottom of the bowl. Continue beating on low speed for 1 to 2 minutes, until the mixture is fully incorporated.

5. Add ½ the eggnog and the vanilla to the bowl of the stand mixer and beat on low speed until the mixture is smooth. Scrape down the sides and bottom of the bowl and add the rum, if using, and the remaining eggnog. Beat on low speed for 1 minute, until the mixture is smooth. The mixture should be well blended, but not overbeaten.

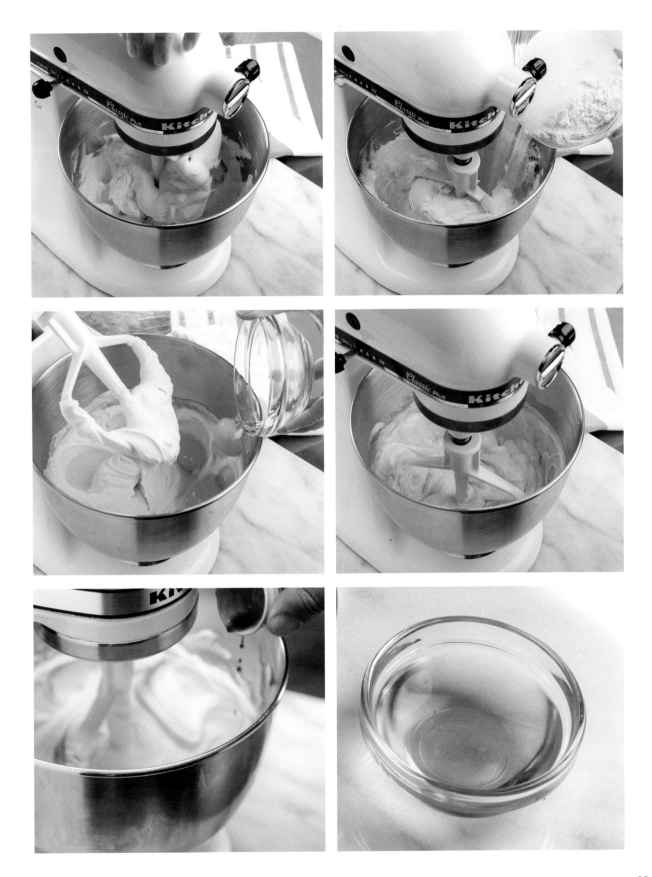

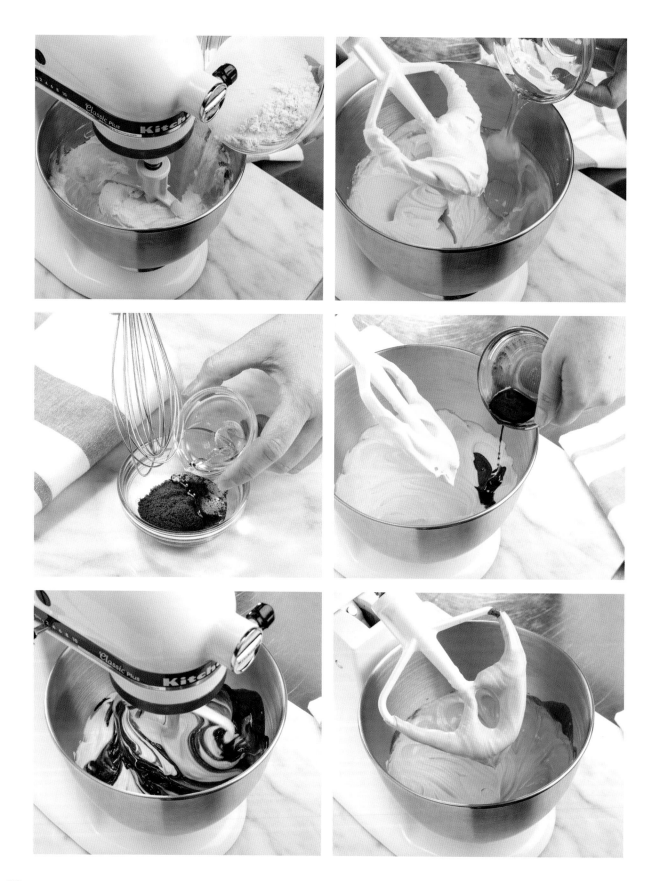

Espresso

YIELD: 25–30 MINI TARTS / 1 (9-INCH) SPRINGFORM CHEESECAKE / 12 SERVINGS

2 (8-ounce) packages cream cheese, room temperature

¾ cup granulated sugar

1 tablespoon cake flour

Pinch salt

1 large whole egg, room temperature

1 large egg yolk, room temperature

2 teaspoons instant coffee or espresso

2 teaspoons boiling water

¼ cup sour cream, room temperature

½ teaspoon vanilla extract

1. In the bowl of a stand mixer fitted with the paddle attachment, beat the cream cheese on medium speed for 2 to 3 minutes, until it is light and fluffy. Scrape down the sides and bottom of the stand mixer bowl to prevent lumps from forming.

2. In a separate medium mixing bowl, combine the sugar, cake flour, and salt. Stir until well combined.

3. Add the contents of the medium mixing bowl to the bowl of the stand mixer and beat on medium speed for 2 to 3 minutes. Scrape down the sides and bottom of the stand mixer bowl and continue beating on medium speed for 1 minute more, until the mixture is smooth and creamy.

4. Reduce the mixer speed to low. Slowly add first the whole egg and then the egg yolk to the bowl, one at a time. After adding each, scrape down the sides and bottom of the bowl. Continue beating on low speed for 1 to 2 minutes, until the mixture is fully incorporated.

5. In a small mixing bowl, combine the instant coffee and boiling water. Stir well, ensuring that the coffee is completely dissolved.

6. Add the contents of the small mixing bowl, the sour cream, and the vanilla to the bowl of the stand mixer and beat on low speed for 1 minute, until the mixture is smooth. Scrape down the sides and bottom of the bowl and beat on low speed for 1 minute more. The mixture should be well blended, but not overbeaten.

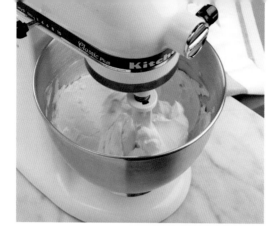

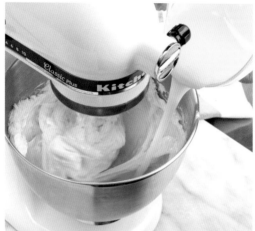

Flan

YIELD: 1 (9-INCH) SPRINGFORM CHEESECAKE /
12 SERVINGS

3 (8-ounce) packages cream cheese, room temperature

14 ounces sweetened condensed milk, divided

1 large whole egg, room temperature

5 large egg yolks, room temperature

1 teaspoon vanilla extract

1. In the bowl of a stand mixer fitted with the paddle attachment, beat the cream cheese on medium speed for 2 to 3 minutes, until it is light and fluffy. Scrape down the sides and bottom of the stand mixer bowl to prevent lumps from forming.

2. Add half of the sweetened condensed milk to the bowl of the stand mixer and beat on low speed for 1 minute. Scrape down the sides and bottom of the stand mixer bowl and continue beating on low speed for 1 minute more, until the mixture is smooth and creamy and free of lumps. Repeat this step with the remaining sweetened condensed milk.

3. Reduce the mixer speed to low. Slowly add first the whole egg and then the egg yolks to the bowl, one at a time. After adding each, scrape down the sides and bottom of the bowl. Continue beating on low speed for 1 to 2 minutes, until the mixture is fully incorporated.

4. Add the vanilla to the bowl of the stand mixer and beat on low speed for 1 minute, until the vanilla is just incorporated into the mixture. The mixture should be well blended, but not overbeaten.

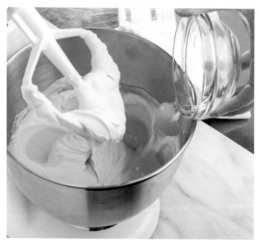

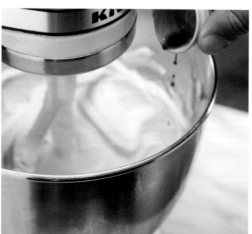

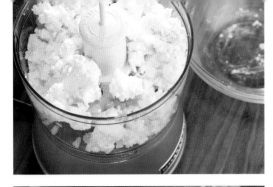

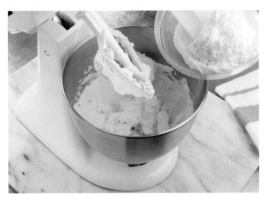

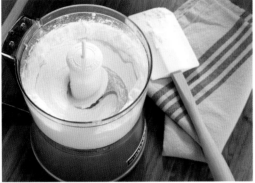

Fresh Cheese

YIELD: 1 (9-INCH) SPRINGFORM CHEESECAKE /
12 SERVINGS

**1/2 cup ricotta cheese, room
temperature**

**6 ounces goat cheese, room
temperature**

**12 ounces cream cheese, room
temperature**

**1/2 cup mascarpone cheese,
room temperature**

**1/2 cup sour cream, room
temperature**

3/4 cup granulated sugar, divided

1 tablespoon cake flour

1 teaspoon lemon zest

**3 large egg whites, room
temperature**

**4 large egg yolks, room
temperature**

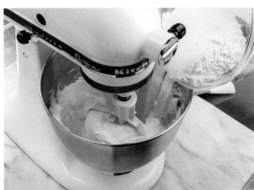

1. In the bowl of a food processor fitted with
   the "S" blade, combine the ricotta and goat
   cheeses and shear them until they are smooth.
   Transfer to a small mixing bowl.

2. In the bowl of a stand mixer fitted with the
   paddle attachment, beat the cream cheese on
   medium speed for 2 to 3 minutes, until it is
   light and fluffy. Scrape down the sides and bottom of the stand mixer bowl to prevent lumps
   from forming and mix for 1 minute more.

3. Add the sheared ricotta and goat cheeses and
   the mascarpone cheese to the bowl of the stand
   mixer and mix on low speed for 1 minute, until
   well blended and smooth. Scrape down the
   sides and bottom of the stand mixer bowl and
   continue beating on low speed for 1 minute
   more, until the mixture is smooth and creamy.

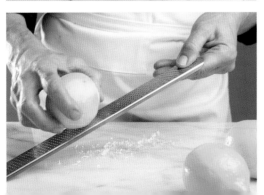

RECIPE CONTINUES ON PAGE 96

4. In a separate medium mixing bowl, combine ½ cup of the sugar with the cake flour. Stir until well combined.

5. Add the contents of the medium mixing bowl to the bowl of the stand mixer and beat on low speed for 1 minute. Scrape down the sides and bottom of the stand mixer bowl and continue beating on low speed for 1 minute more, until the mixture is smooth and creamy.

6. Place the lemon zest on a clean cutting board and sprinkle 1 teaspoon of the granulated sugar over it. Work the sugar into the zest using a spatula or the back of a spoon. Add the sugared zest to the bowl of the stand mixer and beat on low speed for 1 minute, until just combined. Remove the bowl from the stand mixer and set aside.

7. Replace the paddle attachment with the whisk attachment and fit the mixer with a clean, dry bowl. Add the egg yolks and 2 tablespoons of the sugar to the bowl of the stand mixer and whisk for 3 to 4 minutes, until the yolks are light in color and the mixture holds its shape. Transfer the whipped egg yolks to a small mixing bowl, cover with plastic, and set aside.

8. Wash and dry the mixing bowl and whisk attachment. Add the egg whites to the bowl and whisk them for about 2 to 3 minutes, until frothy. Gradually add the remaining 2 tablespoons of the sugar and continue whisking for about 2 minutes, until soft peaks form. Transfer the whipped egg whites to a small mixing bowl, cover with plastic, and set aside.

9. Using a spatula, gently fold the whipped egg yolks into the bowl containing the cheese mixture. Gently mix on low speed until the ingredients are just incorporated. Do not overmix.

10. Using the same spatula, gently fold the whipped egg whites into the bowl containing the cheese mixture. Gently mix on low speed until the ingredients are just incorporated. Do not overmix. The batter should be very light and airy.

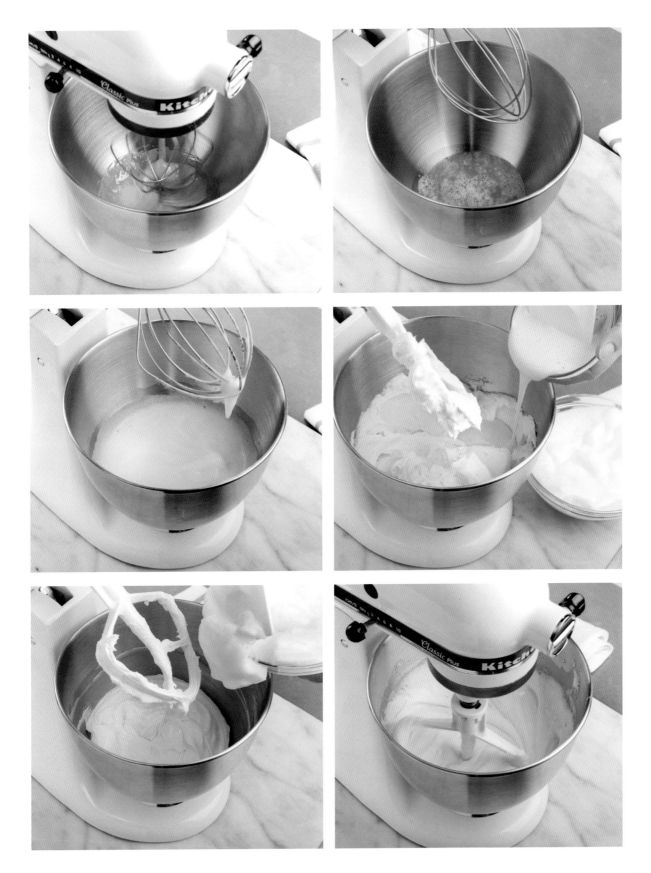

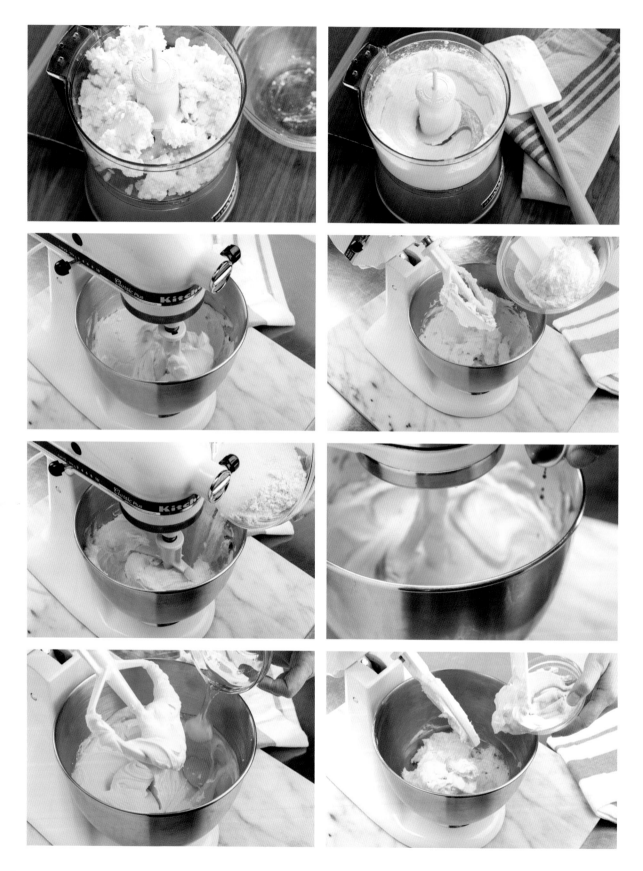

Honey Ricotta

YIELD: 1 (9-INCH) SPRINGFORM CHEESECAKE / 12 SERVINGS

15 ounces ricotta cheese, room temperature

2 (8-ounce) packages cream cheese, room temperature

½ cup granulated sugar

¼ teaspoon salt

2 tablespoons cake flour

¼ cup honey

½ teaspoon vanilla extract

2 large whole eggs, room temperature

½ cup sour cream, room temperature

1. In the bowl of a food processor fitted with the "S" blade, shear the ricotta cheese until it is smooth. Transfer to a small mixing bowl.

2. In the bowl of a stand mixer fitted with the paddle attachment, beat the cream cheese on medium speed for 1 minute, until it is smooth and free of any lumps.

3. Add the sheared ricotta cheese to the bowl of the stand mixer and mix on medium speed for 2 minutes, until well blended and smooth. Scrape down the sides and bottom of the stand mixer bowl to prevent lumps from forming.

4. In a separate medium mixing bowl, combine the sugar, salt, and cake flour. Blend until well combined.

5. Add the contents of the medium mixing bowl to the bowl of the stand mixer and beat on medium speed for 1 to 2 minutes, until smooth.

6. Add the honey and vanilla to the bowl of the stand mixer and beat on low speed for 1 minute, until just combined. Scrape down the sides and bottom of the stand mixer bowl to prevent lumps from forming.

7. Add the eggs, one at a time and scraping down the sides of the bowl as you add them, to the stand mixer bowl and mix on low for 1 to 2 minutes, until the mixture is well combined.

8. Add the sour cream to the bowl of the stand mixer and beat on low speed for 1 minute, until the sour cream is just incorporated into the mixture. The mixture should be well blended, but not overbeaten.

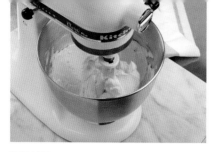

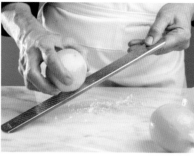

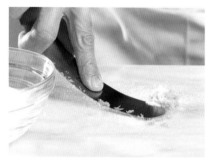

Lemon

YIELD: 1 (9½-INCH × 1-INCH) ROUND TART PAN / 12 SERVINGS

1½ (8-ounce) packages cream cheese, room temperature

1 tablespoon lemon zest

½ cup granulated sugar, divided

½ teaspoon vanilla extract

2 large whole eggs, room temperature

1. In the bowl of a stand mixer fitted with the paddle attachment, beat the cream cheese on medium speed for 1 to 2 minutes, until it is smooth. Scrape down the sides and bottom of the stand mixer bowl to prevent lumps from forming.

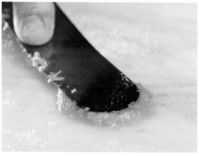

2. Place the lemon zest on a clean cutting board and sprinkle 1 tablespoon of the granulated sugar over it. Work the sugar into the zest using a spatula or the back of a spoon. Add the sugared zest to the bowl of the stand mixer and beat on low speed for 1 minute, until just combined.

3. Add the remaining sugar and the vanilla to the bowl of the stand mixer and beat on low speed for 1 minute, until the mixture is completely blended.

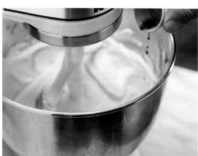

4. Slowly add the eggs to the bowl, one at a time. After adding each, scrape down the sides and bottom of the bowl. Continue beating on low speed for 1 minute, until the mixture is fully incorporated.

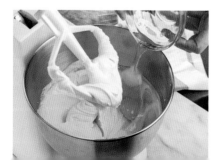

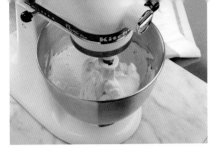

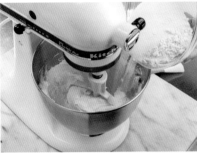

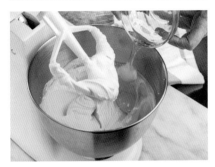

Pumpkin

YIELD: 1 (9¾-INCH × 2-INCH) FLUTED PIE PAN / 12 SERVINGS

3 (8-ounce) packages cream cheese, room temperature

1 cup granulated sugar

¼ cup cake flour

1 teaspoon pumpkin pie spice

¼ teaspoon ground nutmeg

½ teaspoon ground ginger

½ teaspoon salt

2 large whole eggs, room temperature

¾ cup canned pumpkin

⅓ cup sour cream, room temperature

1 teaspoon vanilla extract

1. In the bowl of a stand mixer fitted with the paddle attachment, beat the cream cheese on medium speed for 2 to 3 minutes, until it is light and fluffy. Scrape down the sides and bottom of the stand mixer bowl to prevent lumps from forming.

2. In a separate medium mixing bowl, combine the sugar, cake flour, spices, and salt. Stir until well combined.

3. Add the contents of the medium mixing bowl to the bowl of the stand mixer and beat on medium speed for 1 minute. Scrape down the sides and bottom of the stand mixer bowl and continue beating on medium speed for 1 minute, until the mixture is smooth and creamy.

4. Reduce the mixer speed to low. Slowly add the eggs to the bowl, one at a time. After adding each, scrape down the sides and bottom of the bowl.

5. Add the pumpkin to the bowl of the stand mixer and continue beating on low speed for 1 to 2 minutes, until the mixture is fully incorporated. Scrape down the sides and bottom of the bowl to ensure proper blending.

6. Add the sour cream and the vanilla to the bowl of the stand mixer and beat on low speed for 1 minute, until the mixture is smooth. The mixture should be well blended, but not overbeaten.

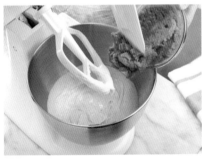

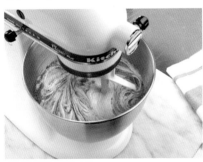

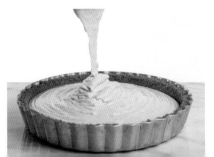

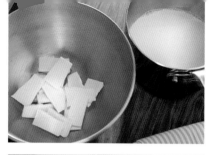
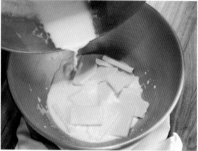
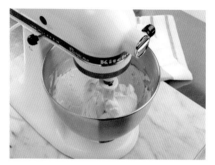
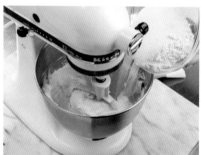
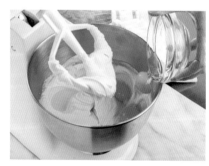

White Chocolate

YIELD: 1 (9-INCH) SPRINGFORM CHEESECAKE /
12 SERVINGS

> 3½ (8-ounce) packages cream cheese, room temperature
>
> 1 cup granulated sugar
>
> 3 tablespoons cake flour
>
> ½ teaspoon salt
>
> 2 large whole eggs, room temperature
>
> 2 large egg yolks, room temperature
>
> 1 recipe White Chocolate Ganache (recipe follows)

1. In the bowl of a stand mixer fitted with the paddle attachment, beat the cream cheese on medium speed for 2 to 3 minutes, until it is light and fluffy. Scrape down the sides and bottom of the stand mixer bowl to prevent lumps from forming.

2. In a separate small mixing bowl, combine the sugar, cake flour, and salt. Stir until well combined.

3. Add the contents of the small mixing bowl to the bowl of the stand mixer and beat on medium speed for 1 to 2 minutes. Scrape down the sides and bottom of the stand mixer bowl and continue beating on medium speed for 1 minute more, until the mixture is smooth and creamy.

4. Reduce the mixer speed to low. Slowly add the eggs and yolks to the bowl, one at a time. After adding each, scrape down the sides and bottom of the bowl. Continue beating on low speed until the mixture is fully incorporated.

5. Add the White Chocolate Ganache to the bowl of the stand mixer and beat on low speed until the mixture is just combined. The mixture should be well blended, but not overbeaten.

VARIATION

White Chocolate and Nutella: Add 1 cup melted Nutella or other hazelnut spread to the batter in spoonfuls. Using a skewer, swirl the Nutella into the batter.

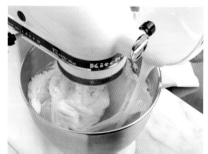

White Chocolate Ganache

YIELD: 9 OUNCES

5 squares (5 ounces) Baker's Premium White Chocolate*
½ cup heavy cream

1. Break the squares of white chocolate into small pieces. Place the white chocolate in a medium heatproof mixing bowl.

2. Place the heavy cream in a small saucepan over medium heat. Cook for 3 to 4 minutes, until a skin begins to form on the cream. Remove from the heat.

3. Transfer the heated cream to the medium mixing bowl containing the white chocolate. Set aside for 1 minute to allow the white chocolate to begin to melt.

4. Stir the mixture vigorously with a silicone spatula, until it is smooth and all the white chocolate has melted. Cover with plastic wrap and set aside.

* White chocolate chips are not recommended for this recipe.

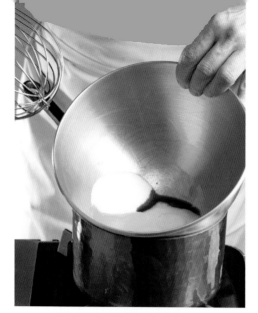

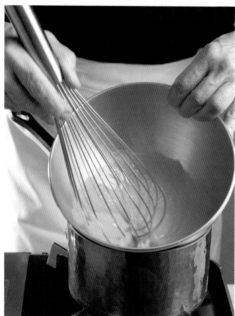

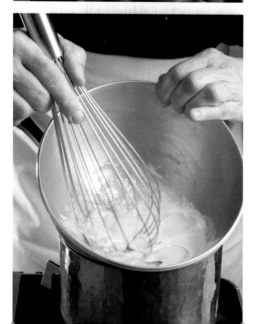

Sabayon

YIELD: 6 INDIVIDUAL (4-INCH) CHEESECAKES / 6 SERVINGS

2 cups water

1 cup granulated sugar, divided

5 large egg yolks, room temperature

4 (8-ounce) packages cream cheese, room temperature

3 tablespoons cake flour

2 large whole eggs, room temperature

¾ cup (6 ounces) sour cream, room temperature

1 teaspoon vanilla extract

1. *Make a sabayon:* Place the 2 cups of water in a saucepan over medium–high heat and bring to a boil. Place a medium heatproof bowl on top of the boiling water and add ½ cup of the sugar and the egg yolks to the bowl. Whisk vigorously until fluffy ribbons form in the mixture and the temperature reaches 150°F. Remove from the heat. Set aside.

2. In the bowl of a stand mixer fitted with the paddle attachment, beat the cream cheese on medium speed for 2 to 3 minutes, until it is smooth and free of lumps.

3. In a separate medium mixing bowl, combine the remaining ½ cup of the sugar and cake flour. Blend until well combined.

4. Resume mixing at medium speed. Gradually add the contents of the medium mixing bowl to the bowl of the stand mixer and beat on medium speed for 2 to 3 minutes, until the mixture is smooth and creamy. Scrape down the sides and bottom of the stand mixer bowl and continue mixing for 1 minute more.

5. Reduce the mixer speed to low. Slowly add the whole eggs to the bowl, one at a time. After adding each, scrape down the sides and bottom of the bowl.

6. Add the sour cream and the vanilla to the bowl of the stand mixer and beat on low speed for 1 minute, until the mixture is smooth. The mixture should be well blended, but not overbeaten.

7. Fold the sabayon into the cream cheese mixture in the bowl of the stand mixer just until incorporated.

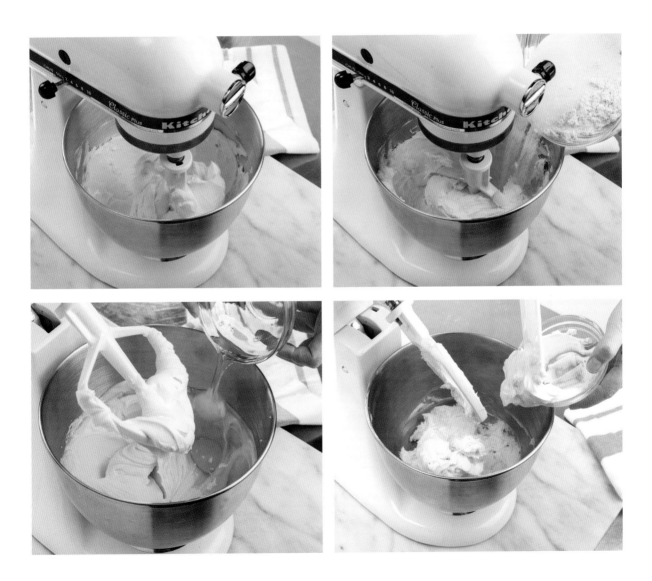

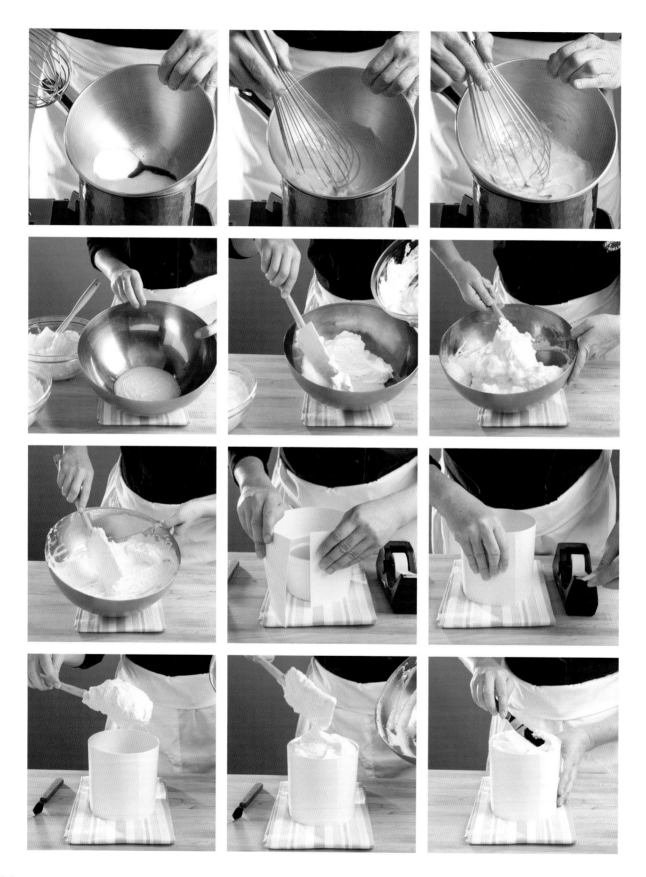

Vanilla Soufflé Glacé

YIELD: 2 (8-INCH) ROUND, DEEP RAMEKINS / 12 SERVINGS

2 cups water
10 large egg yolks, room temperature
1 cup granulated sugar, divided
3 large egg whites, room temperature
2 cups heavy whipping cream, very cold
1 (8-ounce) package mascarpone cheese, room temperature
1 teaspoon vanilla extract
2 whole vanilla beans, split lengthwise

1. *Make a sabayon:* Place the 2 cups of water in a 1-quart saucepan over medium heat and bring to a simmer. Reduce the heat to low and place a medium heatproof bowl on top of the simmering water. Add the egg yolks and ¾ cup of the sugar to the bowl. Whisk vigorously and continuously until the mixture is light and airy. Continue whisking until the sabayon reaches 150°F. Note: Be careful not to curdle the mixture by overheating it or heating it too quickly. Remove from the heat, cover the bowl with plastic wrap, and set aside to cool to room temperature.

2. In the bowl of a stand mixer fitted with the whisk attachment, whip the egg whites on low speed for 2 to 3 minutes, until they are frothy. Slowly add the remaining ¼ cup of sugar to the bowl and continue whipping for 3 to 4 minutes, until soft peaks form.

3. Fit the mixer with a clean, dry bowl that has been chilled in the refrigerator or freezer for 30 minutes or more. Place the very cold heavy whipping cream in the bowl and whip for 3 to 4 minutes, until medium firm peaks form. Watch them carefully and take care not to overwhip the cream.

4. In a separate large mixing bowl, combine the mascarpone cheese and the vanilla extract. Stir until well combined. Using a paring knife, split open the vanilla bean pods and scrape the seeds from the pods. Add the vanilla bean seeds to the mascarpone–vanilla mixture and stir until well combined.

5. Using a spatula, gently fold the sabayon into the bowl containing the mascarpone–vanilla mixture. Gently mix by hand until the ingredients are just incorporated. Do not overmix.

6. Using the same spatula, gently fold the whipped cream into the bowl containing the sabayon–mascarpone mixture until just incorporated. Do not overmix—the more you stir, the less volume your soufflé will have.

7. Using the same spatula, gently fold the whipped egg whites into the bowl containing the sabayon–mascarpone mixture until just incorporated. Do not overmix—the more you stir, the less volume your soufflé will have.

8. *Prepare the ramekins:* Wrap the outside of each ramekin with a tall, measured piece of card stock, as shown in photo. (The card stock should measure about two inches above the rim of the ramekin.) Secure the card stock around each ramekin with several pieces of tape.

9. Carefully divide the mixture evenly between the two ramekins, smoothing the soufflé evenly across the surface. Cover each with plastic wrap. Freeze overnight before serving.

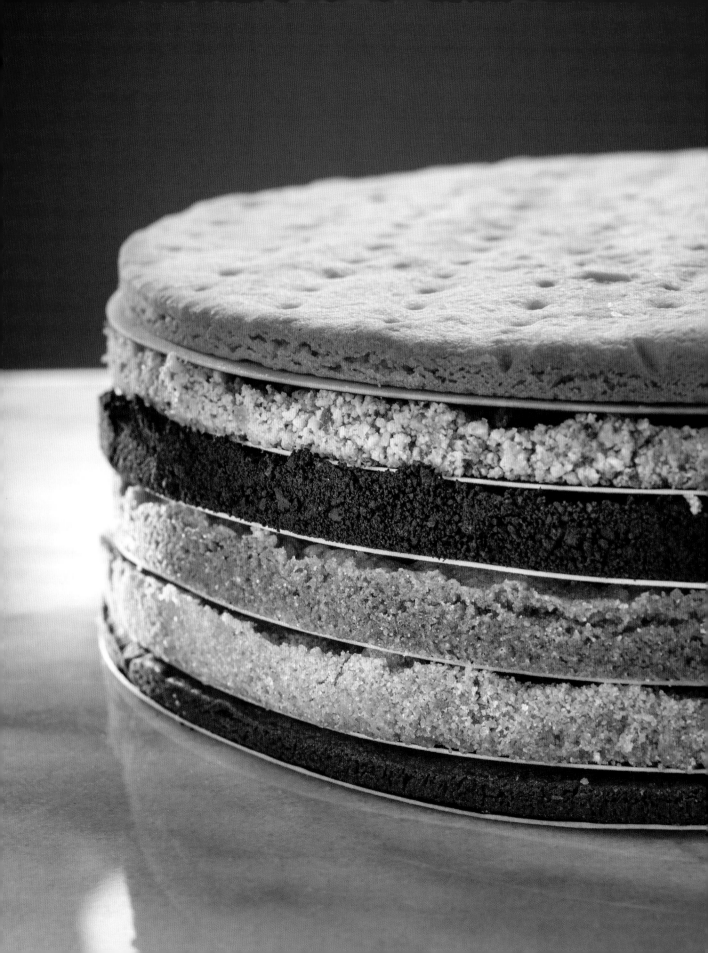

CRUSTS

Shortbread

YIELD: 2 (8- OR 9-INCH) SPRINGFORM BOTTOM CRUSTS, 4 (6-INCH) SPRINGFORM BOTTOM CRUSTS, 1 (9-INCH) TART CRUST WITH CRUST UP THE SIDES, 18 (1½-INCH) TARTLET PANS, 12 (3-INCH) TART PANS

1½ sticks (12 tablespoons) cold unsalted butter

½ cup confectioners' sugar

½ teaspoon salt

¼ teaspoon vanilla extract

1½ cups all-purpose flour

1. In the bowl of a stand mixer fitted with the paddle attachment, cream the butter and confectioners' sugar until the mixture is light and fluffy.

2. Add the salt and vanilla and beat on low speed until the mixture is fully incorporated.

3. Add the flour and beat on low speed until the mixture is fully incorporated and the dough comes together.

4. Shape the dough into a disc. Wrap in plastic and refrigerate for 2 hours.

5. Preheat the oven to 350°F.

6. On a lightly floured surface, roll out the dough to ¼-inch thickness. Use the pan(s) as a template and trim the dough to fit the pan(s).

7. Grease the pan(s). Carefully lay the disc(s) of dough inside the pan(s) and press down, fitting evenly. Using a fork, dock the dough to ensure even baking.

8. Place the pan(s) in the center of the oven, directly on the middle shelf. Bake for 12 to 15 minutes, until golden brown. Remove from the oven and set aside to cool to room temperature, about 1 hour.

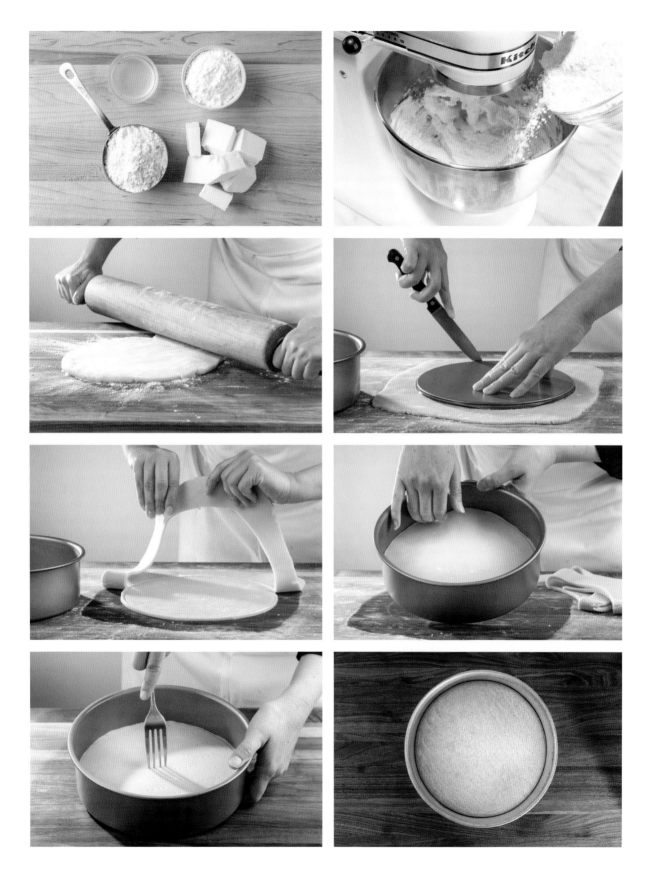

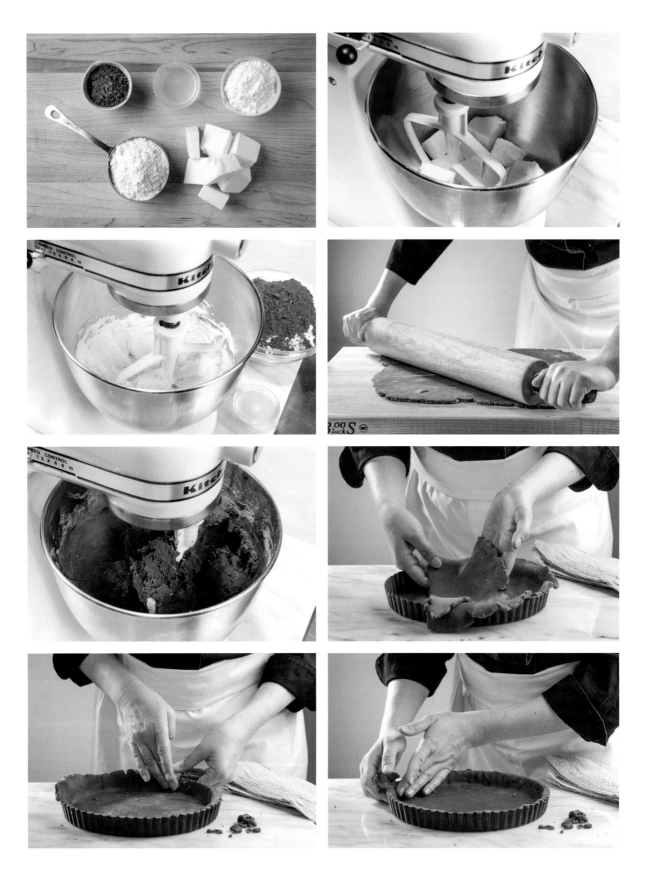

Chocolate Shortbread

YIELD: 2 (8- OR 9-INCH) BOTTOM CRUSTS, 4 (6-INCH) BOTTOM CRUSTS, 1 (9 INCH × 1-INCH) FLUTED TART CRUST WITH CRUST UP THE SIDES, 2 (14-INCH × 4.5-INCH × 1-INCH) LONG RECTANGLE TART CRUSTS WITH CRUST UP THE SIDES, 18 (1½-INCH) TARTLET SHELLS

1½ sticks (12 tablespoons) cold unsalted butter

2/3 cup confectioners' sugar

½ teaspoon salt

¼ teaspoon vanilla extract

1½ cups all-purpose flour

3 tablespoons cocoa powder

1. In the bowl of a stand mixer fitted with the paddle attachment, cream the butter and confectioners' sugar until the mixture is light and fluffy.

2. Add the salt and vanilla to the bowl and beat on low speed until the mixture is fully incorporated.

3. Add the flour and cocoa powder to the bowl and beat on low speed until the mixture is fully incorporated and the dough comes together.

4. Shape the dough into a disc. Wrap in plastic and refrigerate for 2 hours.

5. Preheat the oven to 350°F.

6. On a lightly floured surface, roll out the dough to ¼-inch thickness. Use the pan(s) as a template and trim the dough to fit the pan(s).

7. Grease the pan(s). Carefully lay the disc(s) of dough inside the pan(s) and press down, fitting evenly. Using a fork, dock the dough to ensure even baking.

8. Place the pan(s) in the center of the oven, directly on the middle shelf. Bake for 10 to 12 minutes. Remove from the oven and set aside to cool to room temperature, about 1 hour.

Almond Streusel

YIELD: 2½ CUPS / 10 (2-OUNCE) INDIVIDUAL CRUSTS

½ cup all-purpose flour

¾ cup granulated sugar

5 tablespoons cold unsalted butter

¼ teaspoon salt

¾ cup slivered almonds

1. Preheat the oven to 325°F.

2. In the bowl of a stand mixer fitted with the paddle attachment, combine the flour, sugar, and salt. Beat on low speed until well combined.

3. Using a pastry blender or fork, cut in the butter until the mixture is crumbly. Be careful not to overmix.

4. Using a wooden spoon or silicone spatula, gently stir in the slivered almonds. (It is always best to do this by hand, as the paddle on a mixer will break and crush the almonds.)

5. Line a baking sheet with parchment paper. Crumble the mixture onto the baking sheet and bake for 8 to 10 minutes, until the mixture starts to brown. (Watch it carefully—the streusel should be only lightly toasted.) Remove from the oven and set aside to cool to room temperature, about 1 hour.

Brown Sugar Streusel

YIELD: 1 (9-INCH) SPRINGFORM CHEESECAKE CRUST, 2 (8- AND 9-INCH) BOTTOM CRUSTS, 4 (6-INCH) BOTTOM CRUSTS, 6 (4-INCH) BOTTOM CRUSTS (SEE SABAYON RECIPE ON P. 104), 1 (9-INCH) FLUTED TART CRUST WITH CRUST UP THE SIDES

1 cup all-purpose flour

½ cup light brown sugar

5 tablespoons cold unsalted butter

½ teaspoon ground cinnamon

¼ teaspoon salt

1. Preheat the oven to 350°F.

2. In the bowl of a stand mixer fitted with the paddle attachment, combine the flour, sugar, cinnamon, and salt. Beat on low speed until well combined.

3. Using a pastry blender or fork, cut in the butter until the mixture is crumbly. Be careful not to overmix.

4. Grease the pan(s). Press the mixture into the bottom of the pan(s).

5. To set the crust, bake for 5 minutes. Remove from the oven and set aside to cool to room temperature, about 1 hour.

VARIATION

Toasted Oat and Pecan Streusel: Add ¼ cup lightly toasted oats and ¼ cup chopped pecans in Step 2.

Chocolate Crumb

YIELD: 1 (9-INCH) BOTTOM CRUST

1¹/₂ cups (16 ounces) finely ground chocolate wafer crumbs
¹/₄ cup confectioners' sugar
¹/₄ cup unsalted butter, melted

1. Preheat the oven to 350°F.

2. Place the chocolate wafer crumbs in a large mixing bowl. Using a mesh strainer or sifter, sift the confectioners' sugar into the crumbs. Using your hands, stir the mixture until it is well combined.

3. Add the butter to the crumb mixture. Using your hands, stir the mixture until it is well combined and moistened.

4. Grease the pan(s). Press the mixture into the bottom of the pan(s).

5. To set the crust, place the pan(s) in the center of the oven, directly on the middle shelf. Bake for 8 minutes. Remove from the oven and set aside to cool to room temperature, about 1 hour.

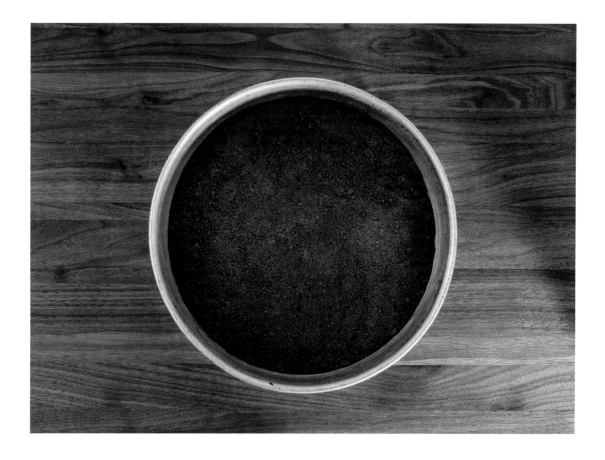

Graham Crumb

YIELD: 2 (8- OR 9-INCH) BOTTOM CRUSTS, 4 (6-INCH) BOTTOM CRUSTS, 1 (9-INCH) FLUTED TART CRUST WITH CRUST UP THE SIDES, 10 INDIVIDUAL (3-INCH) BOTTOM CRUSTS

2 cups (16 ounces) finely ground graham cracker crumbs

¼ cup light brown sugar, firmly packed

¼ cup unsalted butter, melted

1 large egg white

1. Preheat the oven to 350°F.

2. In a medium mixing bowl, combine the graham cracker crumbs and brown sugar. Using your hands, stir the mixture until the crumbs and sugar are completely combined.

3. Add the butter to the crumb mixture. Using your hands, stir the mixture until it is well combined and moistened.

4. In a small mixing bowl, use a fork to lightly whisk the egg white. Add the whisked egg white to the crumb mixture. Using your hands, stir the mixture until it is well combined.

5. Grease the pan(s). Press the mixture into the bottom of the pan(s).

6. To set the crust, place the pan(s) in the center of the oven, directly on the middle shelf. Bake for 8 minutes. Remove from the oven and set aside to cool to room temperature, about 1 hour.

VARIATIONS

Cinnamon Graham Crumb: Add ½ teaspoon ground cinnamon during step 2.

Nutmeg Graham Crumb: Add 1 teaspoon ground nutmeg during step 2.

Toasted Almond

YIELD: 1 (8- OR 9-INCH) BOTTOM CRUST, 2 (6-INCH) BOTTOM CRUSTS, 1 (9-INCH) FLUTED CRUST
WITH CRUST UP THE SIDES

1 cup whole skinned almonds, toasted

2 tablespoons granulated sugar

½ teaspoon salt

1 tablespoon unsalted butter, melted

1. Preheat the oven to 350°F.

2. In the bowl of a food processor fitted with the "S" blade, grind the almonds, sugar, and salt. Process until the mixture becomes moist and crumbly.

3. Add the melted butter and process again until thoroughly combined.

4. Grease the pan(s). Press the mixture into the bottom of the pan(s).

5. To set the crust, bake for 5 minutes. Remove from the oven and set aside to cool to room temperature, about 1 hour.

FINISHING TOUCHES
Chocolates, Caramels, and Compotes

Bittersweet Chocolate Ganache

YIELD: ENOUGH TO COVER 1 (9-INCH) CHEESECAKE

16 ounces bittersweet chocolate

1 cup heavy cream

1. Chop the chocolate into small pieces. Place the chocolate in a medium heatproof mixing bowl.

2. Place the heavy cream in a small saucepan over medium heat. Cook for 3 to 4 minutes, until a skin begins to form on the cream. Remove from the heat.

3. Transfer the heated cream to the medium mixing bowl containing the chocolate. Set aside for 1 minute to allow the chocolate to begin to melt.

4. Whisk the mixture vigorously, until it is smooth and all the chocolate has melted. Use immediately.

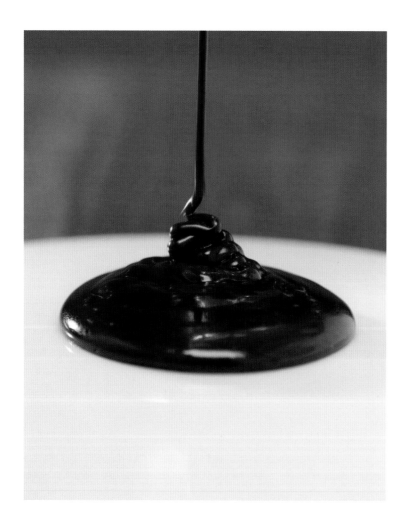

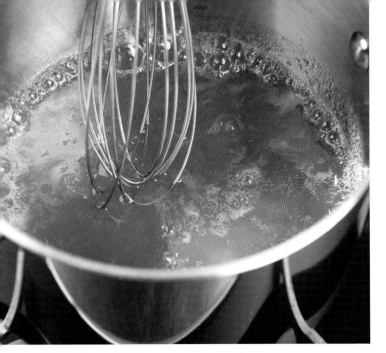

Quick Apricot Glaze

YIELD: ENOUGH TO COVER 1 (9-INCH) CHEESECAKE

8 ounces apricot jam

2 tablespoons water

1. Combine the apricot jam and water in a small saucepan over medium heat. Cook for 2 to 3 minutes, until the jam begins to loosen. Remove from the heat.

2. Using a mesh strainer to filter out any larger pieces of the apricot, transfer the mixture into a small bowl. Cover and refrigerate.

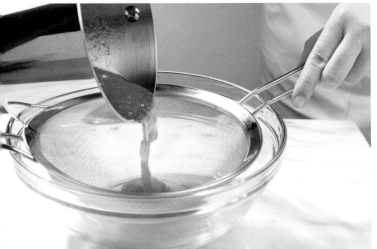

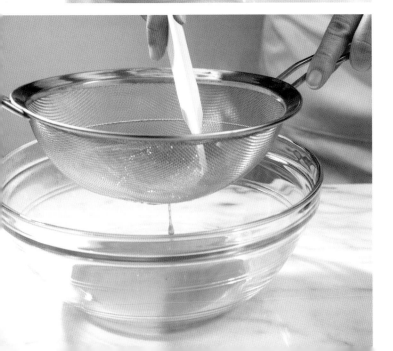

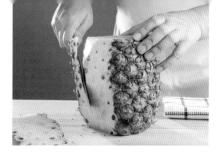

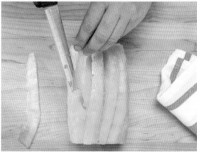

Caramelized Pineapple

YIELD: ENOUGH TO DECORATE 1 (8-INCH) CHEESECAKE

1 fresh whole pineapple
¼ cup unsalted butter, room temperature
½ cup granulated sugar

1. Prepare the pineapple by trimming away its outer skin using a sharp paring knife. Turn the pineapple on its side and cut it lengthwise from top to bottom. Then, cut a second slit right next to the first cut, forming a long, skinny "V" shaped wedge. Once the "V" shaped wedge has been made, remove and discard the wedge. Repeat the process, in the end making 6 wedge cuts in the fruit. This creates a fringed effect on the edges of the pineapple. Do not core the pineapple.

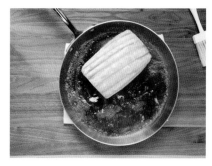

2. In a sauté pan large enough to hold the whole pineapple over medium heat, combine the sugar and butter. Cook for 2 to 4 minutes, until caramelized to a light amber color.

3. Reduce the heat to very low and carefully place the pineapple in the caramel. Cook, turning frequently and basting the caramel syrup over the pineapple, for about 10 minutes, until the caramel has completely saturated the pineapple. Remove from the heat.

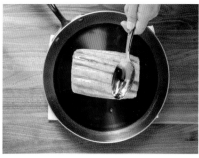

4. Remove the pineapple from the pan and set it aside on a plate to cool.

5. Cut the pineapple into ⅛-inch-wide slices and core each slice using a small, round cookie cutter. Set aside one whole round slice to use as the center piece of each cake and cut the remaining slices in half.

6. Place the pineapple half slices on the cake making an outside circle first, with the ruffled edge of the pineapple slices facing the sides of the pan. Continue placing the slices in concentric circles on the cake, creating a flower shape. Finish with the reserved whole slice of pineapple, creating the cake's center.

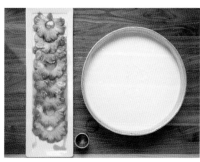

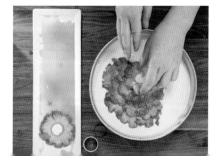

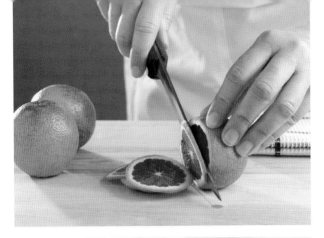

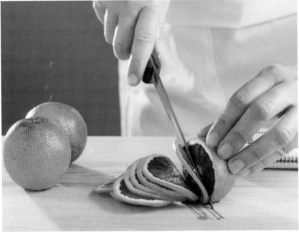

Candied Blood Oranges

YIELD: ENOUGH TO DECORATE 1 (9-INCH) CHEESECAKE

3 blood oranges
1 cup water
1 cup granulated sugar

1. Using a paring knife, thinly slice the blood oranges into ⅛-inch discs.

2. *Make a simple syrup:* Combine the water and sugar in a small saucepan over medium–high heat and bring to a boil.

3. Add the orange slices to the boiling simple syrup, reduce the heat to medium, and allow to simmer for 10 minutes. Remove from the heat and allow the discs to cool in the saucepan.

4. Drain the slices on paper towels. Use immediately or store in an airtight container.

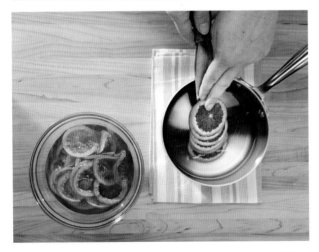

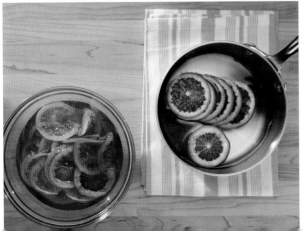

Candied Walnuts

YIELD: ENOUGH TO DECORATE 2 (6-INCH) CHEESECAKES

1 cup water

1 cup granulated sugar

12 ounces walnuts

1. Preheat the oven to 300°F.

2. *Make a simple syrup:* Combine the water and sugar in a small saucepan over medium–high heat and bring to a boil.

3. Add the walnuts to the boiling simple syrup and allow to boil for 5 minutes. Remove from the heat and drain the simple syrup from the saucepan.

4. On a baking sheet lined with parchment paper, evenly spread the walnuts. Place the baking sheet in the center of the oven, directly on the middle shelf. Bake for 20 minutes, stirring the walnuts and rotating the pan 180 degrees halfway through the baking time. When ready, the walnuts will appear shiny and dry. Remove from the oven and set aside to cool to room temperature, about 1 hour.

5. Use immediately or store in an airtight container.

Blackberry Compote

YIELD: 3½ CUPS

3 cups (1½ pints) fresh blackberries, divided
½ cup water
⅓ cup granulated sugar
1½ tablespoons fresh lemon juice

1. In a small saucepan over medium heat, combine 1 cup of the blackberries, water, sugar, and lemon juice and bring to a boil. Boil, stirring frequently, for 3 to 4 minutes, until the sugar is dissolved and the volume has reduced by half. Remove from the heat and set aside to cool to lukewarm.

2. Place the blackberry mixture in a blender and purée. Pour the purée into a fine sieve over a mixing bowl and force it through. Discard any remaining seeds in the sieve.

3. Stir the remaining 2 cups blackberries into the mixture. Mix well and set aside, covered, until ready to use.

Blueberry Compote

YIELD: 2¼ CUPS OR ENOUGH TO TOP 1 (9-INCH) CHEESECAKE

2 cups (15 ounces) fresh blueberries, rinsed, dried, and stems removed
1 recipe Quick Apricot Glaze (see recipe on p. 125), warmed

1. Place the blueberries in a large mixing bowl and pour the warmed Quick Apricot Glaze over them. Mix well and set aside, covered, until ready to use.

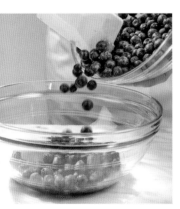
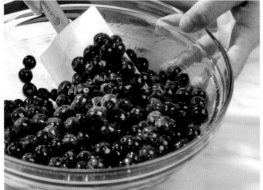
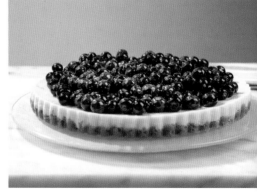

Cherry Compote

YIELD: 3½ CUPS

> **4½ cups (20 ounces) pitted fresh or frozen thawed Bing cherries**
> **1 cup brandy or orange juice**
> **½ cup granulated sugar**

1. In a large, heavy saucepan over medium heat, combine all ingredients and bring to a boil.

2. Reduce the heat to medium–low and simmer, stirring frequently, for 10 minutes, until the cherries have softened and have begun to release their juices. Using a slotted spoon, transfer the cherries to a medium heatproof bowl and set aside.

3. Continue simmering the juices for 15 to 20 minutes, until the mixture is thick enough to coat the back of a spoon. Remove from the heat and pour over the cherries. Mix well and set aside, covered, until ready to use.

Huckleberry Compote

YIELD: 2½ CUPS

> **2½ cups frozen huckleberries**
> **¼ cup granulated sugar**
> **1 tablespoon fresh lemon juice**
> **Zest of 1 lemon**

1. Macerate the frozen huckleberries by placing them in a large mixing bowl and sprinkling the sugar, lemon juice, and zest over them.

2. Toss gently with your hands and cover the bowl with plastic wrap. Place in the refrigerator for 2 hours before using.

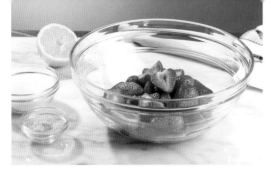

Strawberry Compote

YIELD: 2½ CUPS

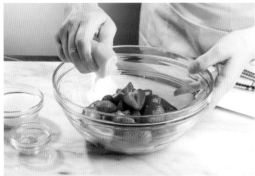

2 cups (14 ounces) whole strawberries, washed, dried, and halved

¼ cup granulated sugar

1 tablespoon fresh lemon juice

Zest of 1 lemon

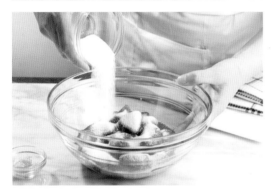

1. Macerate the strawberries by placing them in a large mixing bowl and sprinkling the sugar, lemon juice, and zest over them.

2. Stir well, cover the bowl with plastic wrap, and set aside at room temperature for 2 hours, until the compote has taken on an intense red color and its flavor is very sweet.

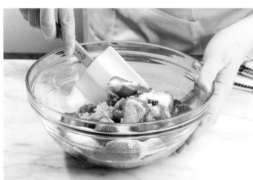

Rhubarb Compote

YIELD: 2¾ CUPS

2 cups (1½ pounds) ½-inch slices fresh rhubarb

¾ cups granulated sugar

1 tablespoon fresh orange juice

1. Combine the rhubarb, sugar, and orange juice in a medium bowl.

2. Cover with plastic wrap and chill in the refrigerator for 1 to 2 days (the longer you macerate the rhubarb, the sweeter it becomes).

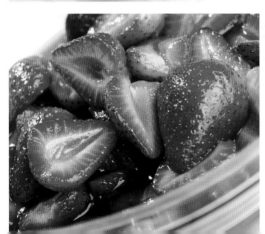

Honey Caramel

YIELD: 2 CUPS OR ENOUGH TO COVER 1 (9-INCH) CHEESECAKE

½ cup honey
⅓ cup granulated sugar
½ tablespoon molasses
¼ teaspoon salt
¼ cup heavy cream

1. In a large, heavy saucepan over medium–high heat, combine all ingredients and bring to a boil. Allow to boil for 1 minute.

2. Reduce the heat to medium and simmer for 5 minutes. Remove from the heat and transfer the caramel to a medium heatproof bowl. Set aside to cool to room temperature for 15 minutes; the caramel will thicken as it cools.

Salted Caramel

YIELD: 2 CUPS OR ENOUGH TO COVER 1 (9-INCH) CHEESECAKE

1 tablespoon corn syrup
2 tablespoons water
¼ teaspoon salt
1 cup granulated sugar
¾ cup heavy cream, warmed to at least 100°F

1. In a heavy 2-quart saucepan over medium heat, combine the corn syrup, water, and salt. Stir with a spatula and cook for 1 minute, until the salt is dissolved and the corn syrup has melted.

2. Sprinkle the sugar into the saucepan, taking care to cover the bottom of the saucepan as evenly as possible. Do NOT stir. Cook, using a pastry brush dipped in water to lightly wash down the sides of the pot, for 3 to 4 minutes, until the mixture begins to caramelize. (Brushing the sides of the pan prevents the formation of sugar crystals.)

3. Once the mixture becomes a light amber color, immediately remove from the heat and add the warmed heavy cream to the saucepan. Stir with a heatproof rubber spatula, scraping the sides and bottom of the pot and making sure to fully incorporate the cream into the caramel, until the mixture is fully combined. *Note: Be careful at this stage, as the caramel is extremely hot and the cream will bubble up and release very hot steam.*

4. Transfer the caramel to a medium heatproof bowl. Set aside to cool to room temperature for 30 minutes; the caramel will thicken as it cools.

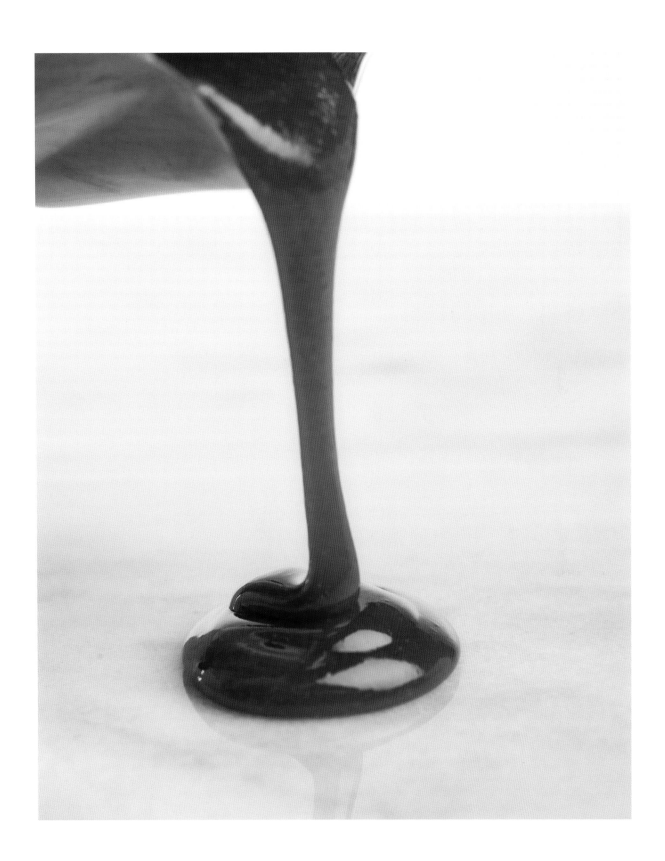

PUTTING IT ALL TOGETHER

Original Plain Cheesecake

Eli's Original Plain Cheesecake is the one that started it all. This simple dessert, made with just a handful of the purest ingredients, set the standard by which all cheesecakes are judged. Eli's Cheesecake is the result of excellent ingredients—including all-natural, slow-cultured dairy products—a long, slow emulsification process, and a rapid baking time in a very hot oven. These elements combine to create its unique flavor, its caramelized top, and its souffléd custard texture. Bon Appetit called Eli's "the best cheesecake for purists." Our Original Plain was a favorite of Frank Sinatra; we regularly sent them to his home in Palm Springs.

Once, we even sent an Original Plain to the Dalai Lama, when he was staying in Washington, DC. We were staying in a hotel room on the same floor, so when our paths crossed, we asked if he liked cheesecake. Sure enough, he did.

YIELD: 1 (9-INCH) SPRINGFORM CHEESECAKE PAN / 12 SERVINGS

Shopping List

FOR THE SHORTBREAD CRUST:

1½ sticks (12 tablespoons) cold unsalted butter

½ cup confectioners' sugar

½ teaspoon salt

¼ teaspoon vanilla extract

1½ cups all-purpose flour

FOR THE ORIGINAL PLAIN BATTER:

4 (8-ounce) packages cream cheese, room temperature

1 cup granulated sugar

¼ cup cake flour

2 large whole eggs, room temperature

1 large egg yolk, room temperature

¾ cup sour cream, room temperature

1 teaspoon vanilla extract

¼ teaspoon salt

RECIPE CONTINUES ON PAGE 133

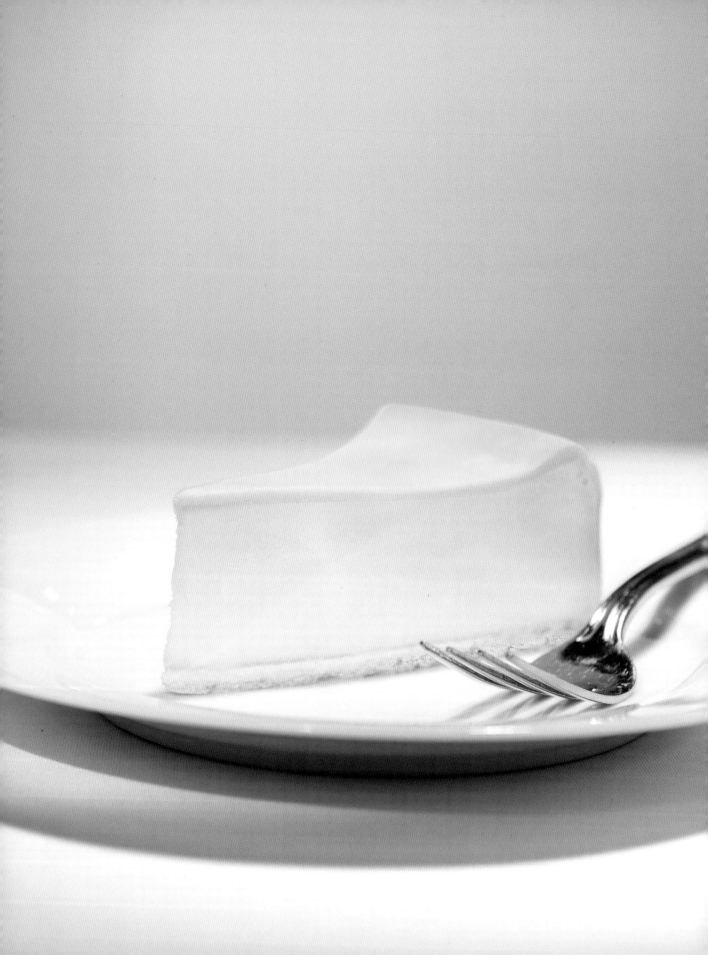

ORIGINAL PLAIN CHEESECAKE *(CONTINUED FROM PAGE 131)*

1. Prepare the Shortbread Crust (see recipe on p. 110) in a 9-inch springform pan. Follow the recipe as directed.

2. Prepare the Original Plain batter (see recipe on p. 78). Follow the recipe as directed.

3. Preheat the oven to 375°F. Generously grease and flour the springform pan (see Trade Secret on p. 76). Fill the springform pan with the Original Plain batter.

4. Place the filled springform pan in the center of the oven, directly on the middle shelf. Bake for 15 minutes, then rotate the cake 180 degrees to ensure even browning. (All ovens bake differently, so be alert for hot spots in your own oven.)

5. Bake for 15 minutes more, and again rotate the cake 180 degrees. The cake should be starting to soufflé and should be light in color. Continue to bake for 10 minutes more, for a total of 40 minutes at 375°F.

6. Reduce the oven temperature to 250°F and leave the oven door slightly ajar. The cake should be golden brown and lightly souffléd on the sides. Leave the cake in the oven for 10 minutes more. (This step and the two that follow allow the cake to cool to room temperature gently, preventing cracking.) Give the cake a gentle shake; it is done if the center of the cake jiggles and the surface of the cake is slightly firm. Turn the oven off and open the oven door wide. Leave the cake in the oven for 10 minutes more. Remove from the oven and set aside to cool to room temperature, about 1 hour.

7. Loosen the cheesecake from the springform pan by sliding an offset spatula around the inside ring. Remove the springform pan from the cake and transfer to a plate. Refrigerate for at least 8 hours or overnight before serving.

8. Transfer to the freezer for 2 to 3 hours before slicing.

9. Slice the cake with a thin, nonserrated knife that is dipped in hot water and wiped dry after each slice. Serve immediately or store in the freezer well wrapped for up to 3 months.

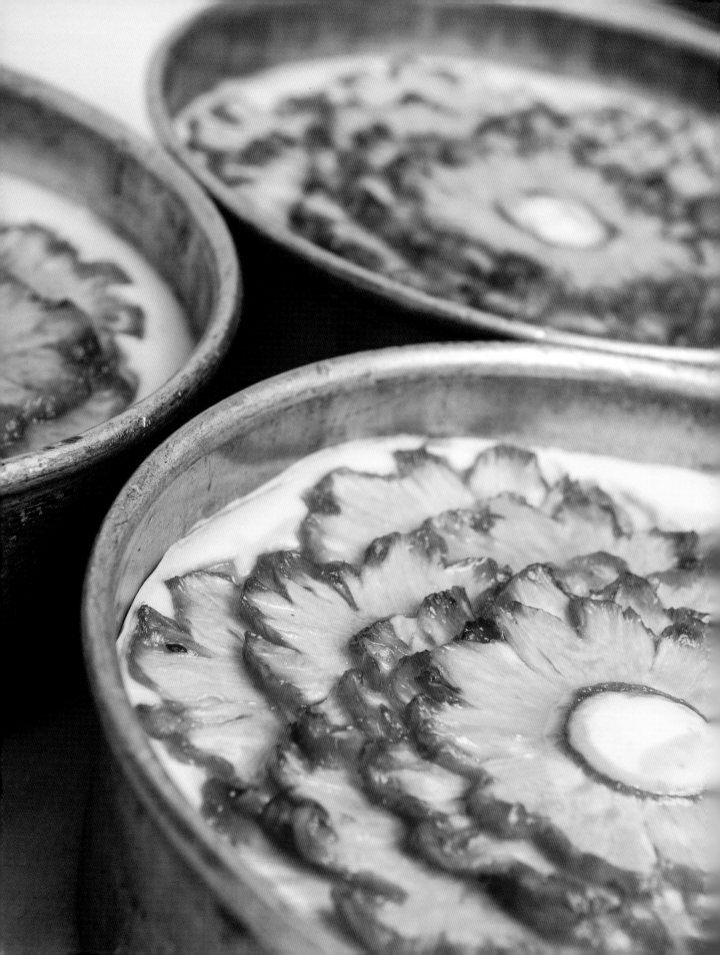

Original Plain Cheesecake with Caramelized Pineapple

YIELD: 1 (8-INCH) SPRINGFORM CHEESECAKE PAN / 12 SERVINGS

Eli's sister Bertha—who was known to all as Aunt Ber—used pineapple in many of the desserts she made. She did them all: pineapple-lined Jell-O molds, pineapple upside down cakes, Hawaiian salad (a concoction of sour cream, Cool Whip, pineapple, coconut, mini marshmallows, and oranges—this was the Sixties, after all). In a nod to Aunt Ber, we've created a caramelized right-side-up tart with a filling of Eli's Original Plain Cheesecake.

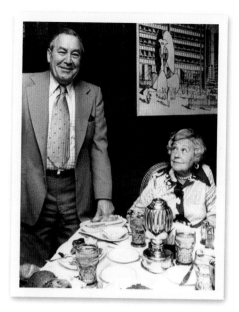

Eli with his sister Bertha at Eli's The Place For Steak.

Shopping List

FOR THE SHORTBREAD CRUST:

1½ sticks (12 tablespoons) cold unsalted butter

½ cup confectioners' sugar

½ teaspoon salt

¼ teaspoon vanilla extract

1½ cups all-purpose flour

FOR THE CARAMELIZED PINEAPPLE:

1 fresh whole pineapple

¼ cup unsalted butter

½ cup granulated sugar

FOR THE ORIGINAL PLAIN BATTER:

4 (8-ounce) packages cream cheese, room temperature

1 cup granulated sugar

¼ cup cake flour

2 large whole eggs, room temperature

1 large egg yolk, room temperature

¾ cup sour cream, room temperature

1 teaspoon vanilla extract

¼ teaspoon salt

RECIPE CONTINUES ON PAGE 136

ORIGINAL PLAIN CHEESECAKE WITH CARAMELIZED PINEAPPLE *(CONTINUED FROM PAGE 135)*

1. Prepare the Shortbread Crust (see recipe on p. 110) in 2 (8-inch) cake pans. Follow the recipe as directed.

2. Prepare the Caramelized Pineapple (see recipe on p. 122). Follow the recipe as directed.

3. Prepare the Original Plain batter (see recipe on p. 78). Follow the recipe as directed.

4. Preheat the oven to 325°F. Divide the Original Plain batter evenly among the 2 cake pans. Generously grease and flour the springform pan (see Trade Secret on p. 76). Place the 2 full circles of pineapple in the center of each cake and arrange the remaining slices in concentric rings starting around the outer edge and working toward the center.

5. Place the filled cake pans in the center of the oven, directly on the middle shelf. Bake for 20 minutes.

6. Reduce the oven temperature to 200°F. Leave the cake pans in the oven for 30 minutes more, until both cakes jiggle slightly in the center. (This step allows the cheesecake to continue cooking slowly and gently, preventing cracking.) Remove from the oven and set aside to cool to room temperature, about 1 hour.

7. Loosen the springform rings from the pans by sliding an offset spatula around the inside of each pan. Remove the springform rings and transfer the cakes, with the pan bottoms still in place, to plates. Using a pastry brush, finish the tarts by gently brushing the pineapple with the reserved caramel. Refrigerate for at least 8 hours or overnight before serving.

8. Transfer the cheesecake to serving plates and place in the freezer for 2 to 3 hours before slicing.

9. Slice the cheesecake with a thin, nonserrated knife that is dipped in hot water and wiped dry after each slice. Serve immediately or store in the freezer well wrapped for up to 3 months.

ELI'S TRADE SECRET *Always use a serrated knife when cutting the pineapple; you'll have much more control.*

Original Plain Cheesecake with Strawberry Compote

YIELD: 1 (9-INCH) SPRINGFORM CHEESECAKE PAN / 12 SERVINGS

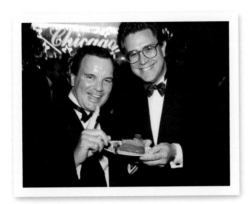

Marc and Mayor Daley at the inauguration.

Mayor Richard M. Daley was always there for Eli's and the Schulman family during his 22-year tenure as Mayor of Chicago. We made a giant cheesecake for his first inauguration in 1989, and he was a part of all the important events in The Eli's Cheesecake Company's history—the dedication of the Eli M. Schulman Playground at Seneca Park in 1990; the opening of Eli's Cheesecake World in 1996 (he was instrumental in getting the land and financing to build it in Chicago); and our 25th birthday at the 2005 Taste of Chicago. Mayor Daley cared deeply about Chicago's family businesses. Our success would not have been possible without his leadership. We are very pleased that he's a fan of Eli's cheesecake, and strawberry is his personal favorite.

Shopping List

FOR THE SHORTBREAD CRUST:

1½ sticks (12 tablespoons) cold unsalted butter

½ cup confectioners' sugar

½ teaspoon salt

¼ teaspoon vanilla extract

1½ cups all-purpose flour

FOR THE STRAWBERRY COMPOTE:

2 cups (14 ounces) whole strawberries

¼ cup granulated sugar

1 tablespoon fresh lemon juice

Zest of 1 lemon

FOR THE ORIGINAL PLAIN BATTER:

4 (8-ounce) packages cream cheese, room temperature

1 cup granulated sugar

¼ cup cake flour

2 large whole eggs, room temperature

1 large egg yolk, room temperature

¾ cup sour cream, room temperature

1 teaspoon vanilla extract

¼ teaspoon salt

RECIPE CONTINUES ON PAGE 138

ORIGINAL PLAIN CHEESECAKE WITH STRAWBERRY COMPOTE *(CONTINUED FROM PAGE 137)*

1. Prepare the Shortbread Crust (see recipe on p. 110) in a 9-inch springform pan. Follow the recipe as directed.

2. Prepare the Strawberry Compote (see recipe on p. 127). Follow the recipe as directed and store in the refrigerator.

3. Prepare the Original Plain batter (see recipe on p. 78). Follow the recipe as directed.

4. Preheat the oven to 375°F. Generously grease and flour the springform pan (see Trade Secret on p. 76). Fill the springform pan with the Original Plain batter.

5. Place the filled springform pan in the center of the oven, directly on the middle shelf. Bake for 15 minutes, then rotate the cake 180 degrees to ensure even browning. (All ovens bake differently, so be alert for hot spots in your own oven.)

6. Bake for 15 minutes more, and again rotate the cake 180 degrees. The cake should be starting to soufflé and should be light in color. Continue to bake for 10 minutes more, for a total of 40 minutes at 375°F.

7. Reduce the oven temperature to 250°F and leave the oven door slightly ajar. The cake should be golden brown and lightly souffléd on the sides. Leave the cake in the oven for 10 minutes more. (This step and the two that follow allow the cake to cool to room temperature gently, preventing cracking.) Give the cake a gentle shake; it is done if the center of the cake jiggles and the surface of the cake is slightly firm. Turn the oven off and open the oven door wide. Leave the cake in the oven for 10 minutes more. Remove from the oven and set aside to cool to room temperature, about 1 hour.

8. Loosen the cheesecake from the springform pan by sliding an offset spatula around the inside ring. Remove the springform pan from the cake and transfer to a plate. Refrigerate for at least 8 hours or overnight before serving.

9. Transfer to the freezer for 2 to 3 hours before slicing.

10. Slice the cake with a thin, nonserrated knife that is dipped in hot water and wiped dry after each slice. Serve immediately with the Strawberry Compote or store in the freezer well wrapped for up to 3 months.

ELI'S TRADE SECRET

Want to make your strawberry cheesecake a little more interesting? Add chopped fresh basil to the strawberries in the Strawberry Compote (see recipe on p. 127) after they're macerated, right before you serve.

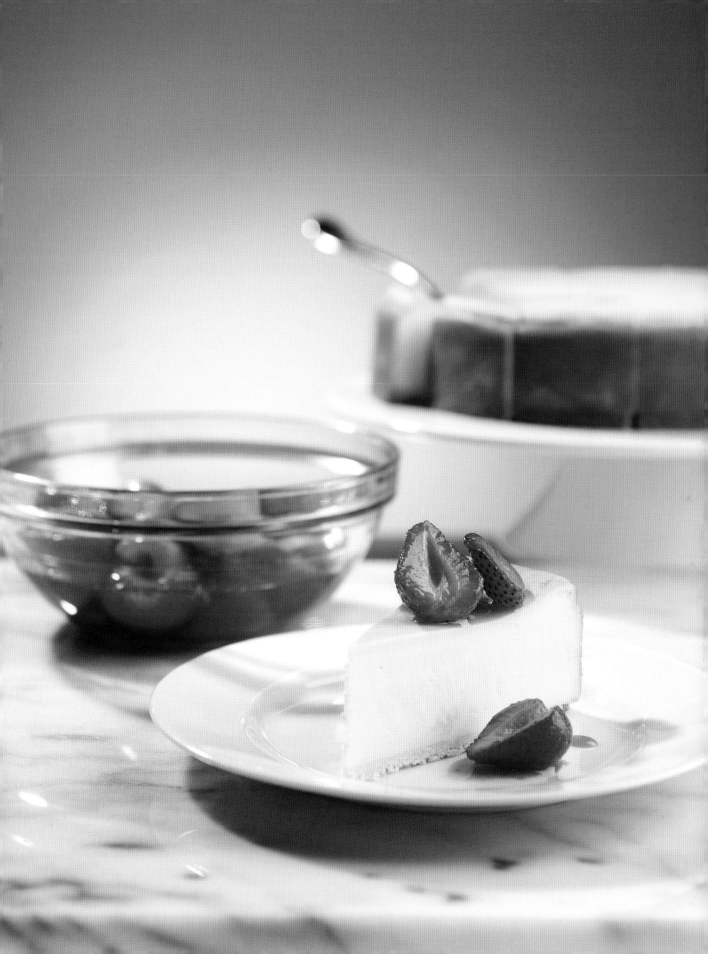

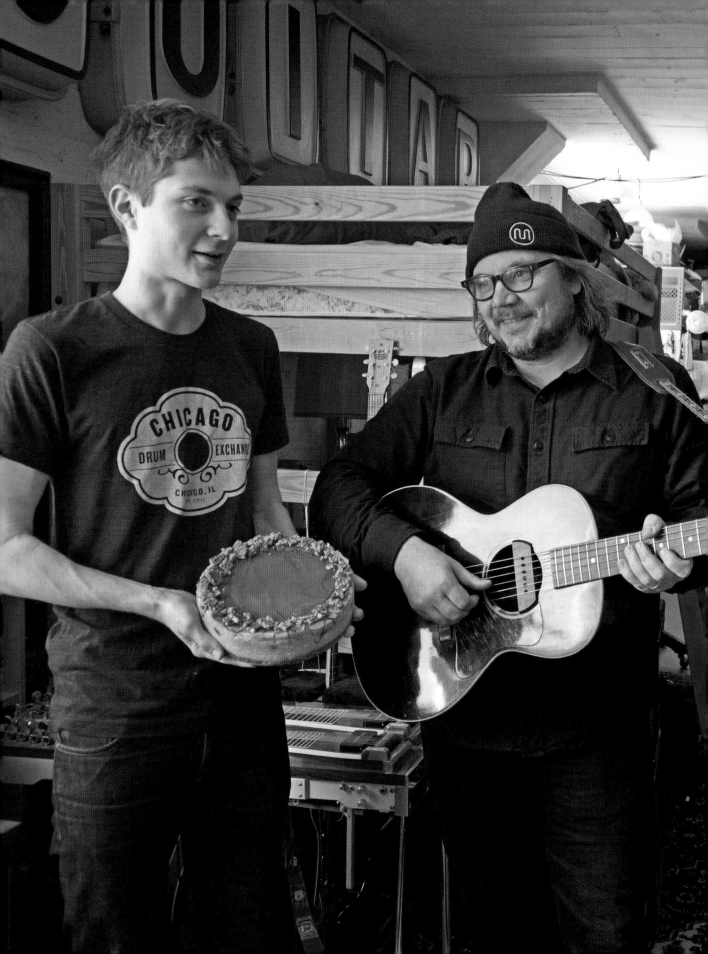

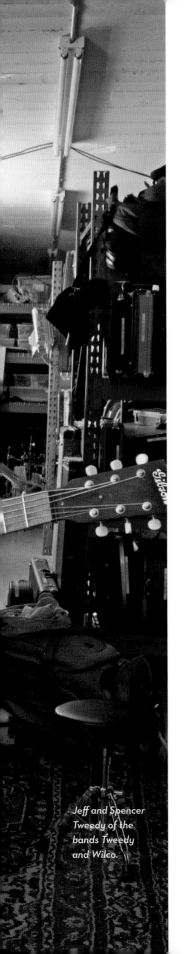

Original Plain Cheesecake with Stroopwafel

YIELD: 1 (9-INCH) SPRINGFORM CHEESECAKE PAN / 12 SERVINGS

Jeff and Spencer Tweedy, of the bands Tweedy and Wilco: "The world is kind of overdue for a stroopwafel cheesecake," said Jeff about his and son Spencer's ultimate cheesecake creation. They based their idea on Susan Tweedy's (Jeff's wife, Spencer's mom) favorite cookie. We love Jeff Tweedy because, like Eli's, Jeff is a symbol of Chicago and maintained his home here while becoming nationally and internationally acclaimed.

Shopping List

FOR THE SHORTBREAD CRUST:

1½ sticks (12 tablespoons) cold unsalted butter

½ cup confectioners' sugar

½ teaspoon salt

¼ teaspoon vanilla extract

1½ cups all-purpose flour

FOR THE ORIGINAL PLAIN BATTER:

4 (8-ounce) packages cream cheese, room temperature

1 cup granulated sugar

¼ cup cake flour

2 large whole eggs, room temperature

1 large egg yolk, room temperature

¾ cup sour cream, room temperature

1 teaspoon vanilla extract

¼ teaspoon salt

2 (6-ounce) packages stroopwafel cookies, cut into small pieces, divided

FOR THE SALTED CARAMEL:

1 tablespoon corn syrup

2 tablespoons water

¼ teaspoon salt

1 cup granulated sugar

¾ cup heavy cream, warmed to at least 100°F

RECIPE CONTINUES ON PAGE 142

ORIGINAL PLAIN CHEESECAKE WITH STROOPWAFEL *(CONTINUED FROM PAGE 141)*

1. Prepare the Shortbread Crust (see recipe on p. 110) in a 9-inch springform pan. Follow the recipe as directed.

2. Prepare the Original Plain batter (see recipe on p. 78). Follow the recipe as directed.

3. Preheat the oven to 325°F. Generously grease and flour the springform pan (see Trade Secret on p. 76). Fill the springform pan with ½ the Original Plain batter. Using an offset spatula, smooth down the batter and sprinkle with ½ the stroopwafel cookie pieces. Carefully deposit the remaining cheesecake batter over the cookie pieces by placing small spoonfuls of batter evenly over the top and then using the offset spatula to smooth the surface.

4. Place the filled springform pan in the center of the oven, directly on the middle shelf. Bake for 40–45 minutes. Give the cake a gentle shake; it is done if the center of the cake jiggles and the surface of the cake is slightly firm. Turn the oven off and open the oven door wide. Leave the cake in the oven for 10 minutes more. Remove from the oven and set aside to cool to room temperature, about 1 hour.

5. Loosen the cheesecake from the springform pan by sliding an offset spatula around the inside ring. Remove the springform pan from the cake and transfer to a plate. Refrigerate for at least 8 hours or overnight before serving.

6. Prepare the Salted Caramel (see recipe on p. 128). Set aside while still warm, but not hot.

7. Pour the Salted Caramel on the center of the cake. Using a wooden spoon or silicone spatula, spread the caramel evenly over the top of the cake, leaving the outer ½ inch of the cake uncoated.

8. While the caramel is still warm, press the remaining stroopwafel cookie pieces into the mostly uncoated area on the outer edge of the cake. Work quickly! As caramel cools, it becomes less sticky and the decorations do not adhere as well.

9. Transfer to the freezer for 2 to 3 hours before slicing.

10. Slice the cake with a thin, nonserrated knife that is dipped in hot water and wiped dry after each slice. Serve immediately or store in the freezer well wrapped for up to 3 months.

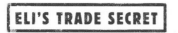 *Stroopwafel cookies come in many flavors. Try something different, such as maple or cinnamon, to add a little more complexity to your cheesecake.*

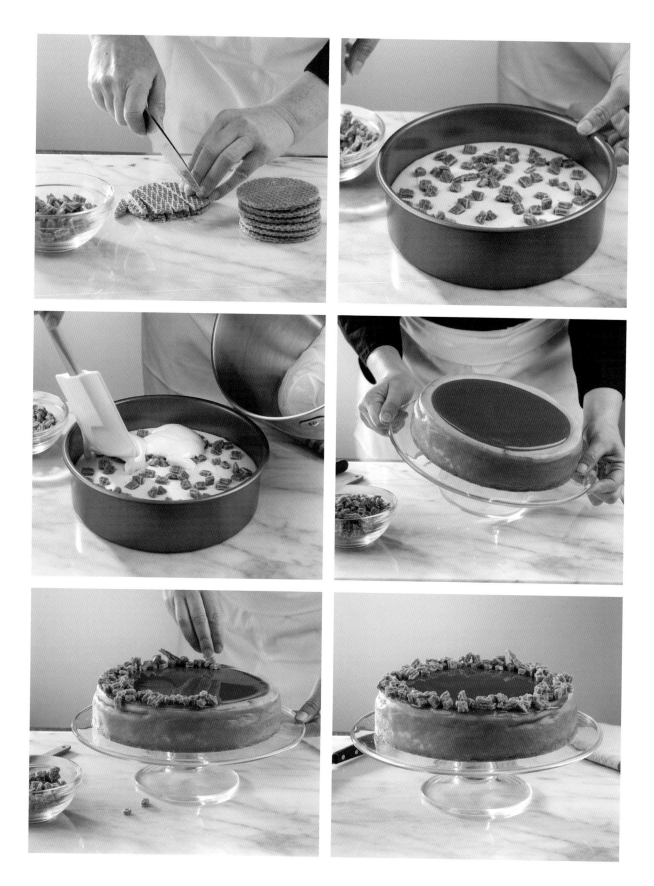

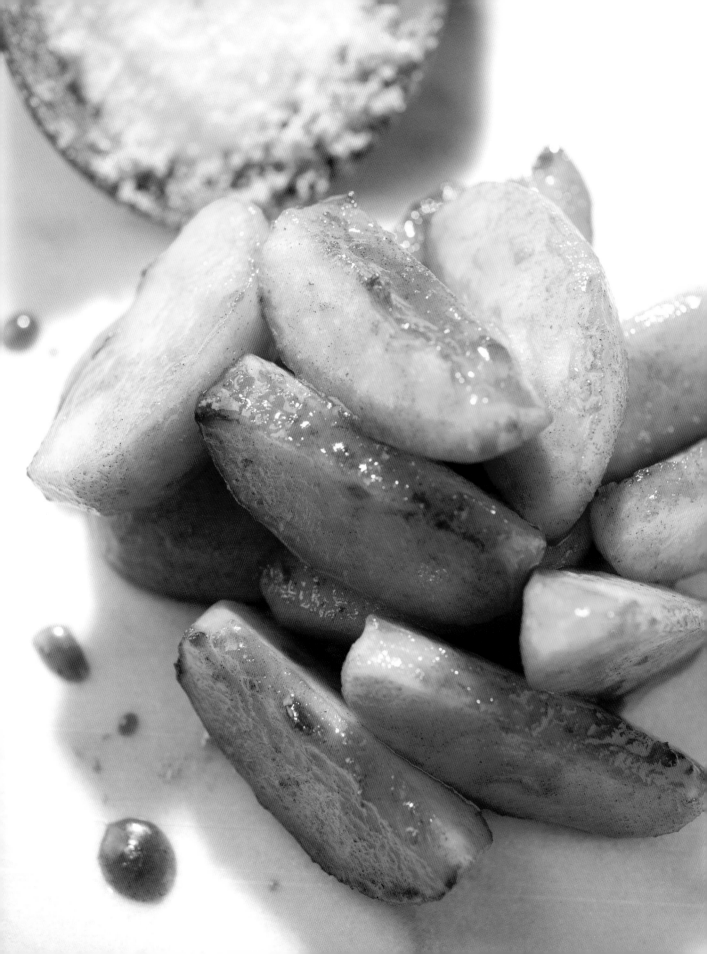

Baked Apple Cheesecake with Toasted Oat and Pecan Streusel

YIELD: 1 (9-INCH) SPRINGFORM CHEESECAKE PAN / 12 SERVINGS

Michigan's Sill Farms, family owned for three generations now, has supplied Eli's Cheesecake with fresh Ida Red apples for more than 20 years. The farm stores apples in sealed, temperature-controlled rooms that keep them as fresh as the day they were picked, enabling us to make cheesecakes with fresh apples year-round.

We asked our good friends Coach Mike Ditka and his wife, Diana, to come up with the "touchdown of cheesecakes." So here it is: Baked Apple Cheesecake with Toasted Oat and Pecan Streusel and plenty of nuts and raisins.

Marc recalls, "The Bears and my dad go way back. Eli personally delivered corned beef sandwiches to legendary sportscasters Jack Brickhouse and Irv Kupcinet every Sunday for 20 years during their radio broadcasts covering the Bears—first at Wrigley Field and then Soldier Field. In the late '60s, Eli also became close friends with Bears' running backs Gayle Sayers and Brian Piccolo. Later, when Brian became sick, Eli and Bears Chairman Ed McCaskey traveled to New York to visit him.

"Coach Ditka and Diana dined at Eli's The Place For Steak after every home game until he opened his own restaurant, Ditka's. In 1986, we were especially proud that the Coach chose Eli's The Place For Steak to celebrate the Bears' win against the Los Angeles Rams that sent them to the Super Bowl. Mayor Harold Washington served Eli's cheesecake at Chicago's Super Bowl party in New Orleans and announced it by name on national television."

RECIPE CONTINUES ON PAGE 146

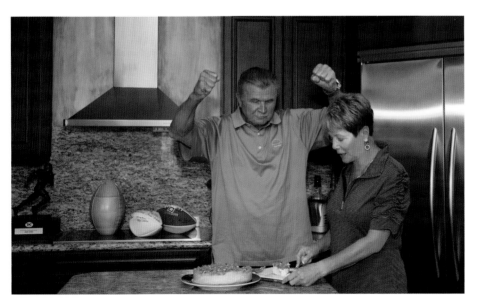

Coach Mike Ditka and his wife, Diana, with the Baked Apple Cheesecake with Toasted Oat and Pecan Streusel

PHOTO BY MICHELLE REED

BAKED APPLE CHEESECAKE WITH TOASTED OAT AND PECAN STREUSEL (CONTINUED FROM PAGE 145)

Shopping List

FOR THE TOASTED OAT AND PECAN STREUSEL:

1 cup all-purpose flour

½ cup light brown sugar

5 tablespoons cold unsalted butter

½ teaspoon ground cinnamon

¼ teaspoon salt

¼ cup lightly toasted oats

¼ cup chopped pecans

FOR THE APPLES:

6 baking (Ida Red or Northern Spy) apples, peeled, cored, and cut into 1-inch-thick wedges

¼ cup granulated sugar

¼ cup light brown sugar

1 teaspoon ground cinnamon

2 tablespoons unsalted butter

FOR THE BAKED APPLE BATTER:

4 (8-ounce) packages cream cheese, room temperature

1 cup granulated sugar

¼ cup cake flour

¼ teaspoon salt

2 large whole eggs, room temperature

1 large egg yolk, room temperature

¾ cup sour cream, room temperature

1 teaspoon vanilla extract

RECIPE CONTINUES ON PAGE 148

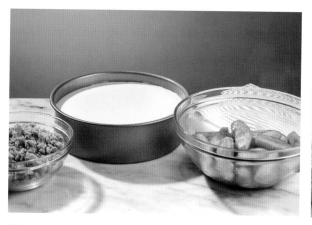
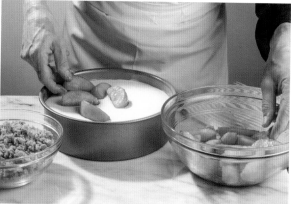

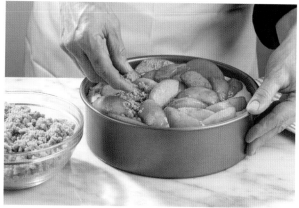
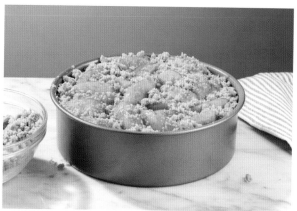

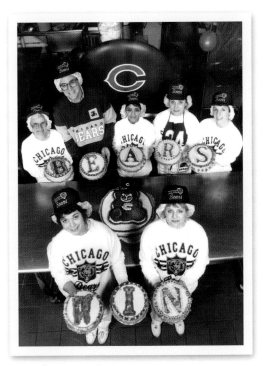

Bears pep rally for the Super Bowl, 1986.

BEAR WITH THEM, they have Super Bowl fever! "Running a temperature" are (standing from left) Mike Ditka, Eli Schulman, (seated from left) Jimmy the Greek and Bears' General Manager Jerry Vainisi. They met to celebrate the Bears' victory Sunday at Eli's Place for Steaks and to plan strategy for Jan. 26 over steaks, ribs and cheesecake.

BAKED APPLE CHEESECAKE WITH TOASTED OAT AND PECAN STREUSEL (CONTINUED FROM PAGE 146)

1. Preheat the oven to 375°F.

2. Prepare the Toasted Oat and Pecan Streusel (see recipe variation on p. 115). Generously grease and flour the springform pan (see Trade Secret on p. 76). Place ⅔ of the mixture in the bottom of a 9-inch springform pan and reserve the other ⅓. Follow the recipe as directed.

3. Place the filled springform pan in the center of the oven, directly on the middle shelf. Bake for 15 minutes. Remove from the oven and set aside to cool to room temperature for 1 hour.

4. Prepare the Baked Apple batter (see recipe on pp. 79). Follow the recipe as directed.

5. Fill the springform pan with the Original Plain batter and top with the Baked Apples. Place the remaining ⅓ of the Streusel Crust mixture on top.

6. Place the filled springform pan in the center of the oven, directly on the middle shelf. Bake for 15 minutes, then rotate the cake 180 degrees to ensure even browning. (All ovens bake differently, so be alert for hot spots in your own oven.)

7. Bake for 15 minutes more, and again rotate the cake 180 degrees. The cake should be starting to soufflé and should be light in color. Continue to bake for 10 minutes more, for a total of 40 minutes at 375°F.

8. Reduce the oven temperature to 250°F and leave the oven door slightly ajar. The cake should be golden brown and lightly souffléd on the sides. Leave the cake in the oven for 10 minutes more. (This step and the two that follow allow the cake to cool to room temperature gently, preventing cracking.) Give the cake a gentle shake; it is done if the center of the cake jiggles and the surface of the cake is slightly firm. Turn the oven off and open the oven door wide. Leave the cake in the oven for 10 minutes more. Remove from the oven and set aside to cool to room temperature, about 1 hour.

9. Loosen the cheesecake from the springform pan by sliding an offset spatula around the inside ring. Remove the springform pan from the cake and transfer to a plate. Refrigerate for at least 8 hours or overnight before serving.

10. Transfer to the freezer for 2 to 3 hours before slicing.

11. Slice the cake with a thin, nonserrated knife that is dipped in hot water and wiped dry after each slice. Serve immediately or store in the freezer well wrapped for up to 3 months.

ELI'S TRADE SECRET *Ida Red and Northern Spy apples are great choices for baking.*

Banana Cheesecake with Bittersweet Ganache

YIELD: 2 (6-INCH) SPRINGFORM CHEESECAKE PANS / 12 SERVINGS

Chocolate and banana is one of the greatest flavor combinations of all time. Our daughters get motivated to make chocolate chip–banana bread whenever they walk by the kitchen counter and spot some overripe bananas. In fact, it was Kori's idea to come up with a banana and chocolate cheesecake recipe in the first place.

Shopping List

FOR THE CHOCOLATE SHORTBREAD CRUST:

1½ sticks (12 tablespoons) cold unsalted butter

2/3 cup confectioners' sugar

1/2 teaspoon salt

1/4 teaspoon vanilla extract

1½ cups all-purpose flour

3 tablespoons cocoa powder

FOR THE BANANA BATTER:

2 (8-ounce) packages cream cheese, room temperature

3/4 cup light brown sugar

2 tablespoons cake flour

2 large whole eggs, room temperature

2 large ripe bananas, puréed (should yield 1 cup)

1/2 teaspoon vanilla extract

1/4 cup sour cream, room temperature

FOR THE BITTERSWEET CHOCOLATE GANACHE:

16 ounces bittersweet chocolate

1 cup heavy cream

RECIPE CONTINUES ON PAGE 151

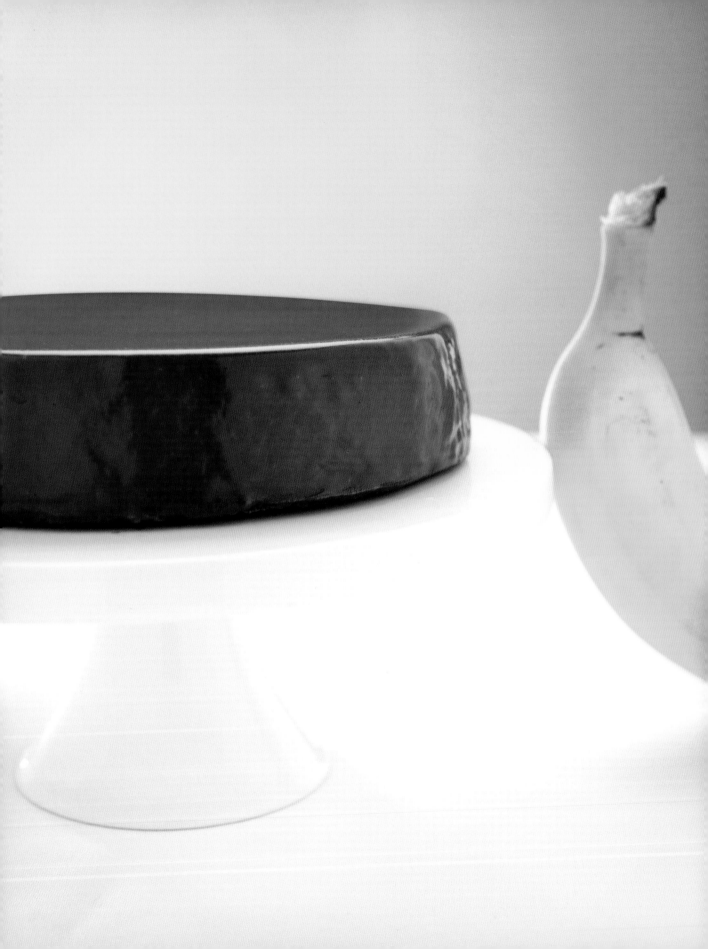

BANANA CHEESECAKE WITH
BITTERSWEET GANACHE *(CONTINUED FROM PAGE 149)*

1. Prepare the Chocolate Shortbread Crust (see recipe on p. 113) in 2 (6-inch) springform pans. Follow the recipe as directed. Roll out the dough in a rectangular shape to ¼-inch thick. Cut out 2 (6-inch) discs of dough and carefully place them in the bottoms of 2 greased (6-inch) springform pans.

2. Prepare the Bittersweet Chocolate Ganache and then the Banana batter (see recipes on pp. 120 and 81, respectively). Follow the recipes as directed.

3. Preheat the oven to 280°F. Generously grease and flour the springform pan (see Trade Secret on p. 76). Pour the Banana batter into the prepared springform pans. Using an offset spatula, smooth down the batter until it is level.

4. Set the springform pans on a baking sheet and place the baking sheet in the center of the oven, directly on the middle shelf. Bake for 30 to 35 minutes, until the cakes are slightly firm to the touch, jiggle in the center, and are lightly souffléd on the sides. (If at the end of this baking time, the cakes are starting to soufflé but still have loose centers, reduce the oven temperature to 200°F and bake for another 5 minutes.) Remove from the oven and set aside to cool to room temperature, about 1 hour.

5. Loosen the cheesecakes from the springform pans by sliding an offset spatula around the inside rings. Remove the springform pans from the cakes and transfer to plates. Refrigerate for 4 hours or overnight to completely set.

6. Prepare the Bittersweet Chocolate Ganache and pour it over the chilled cheesecake, enrobing it completely. Use an offset spatula to evenly spread the ganache.

7. Place the cheesecake in the freezer for 2 to 3 hours before slicing.

8. Slice the cake with a thin, nonserrated knife that is dipped in hot water and wiped dry after each slice. Serve immediately or store in the freezer well wrapped for up to 3 months.

ELI'S TRADE SECRET *The riper the banana, the more intense the banana flavor will be.*

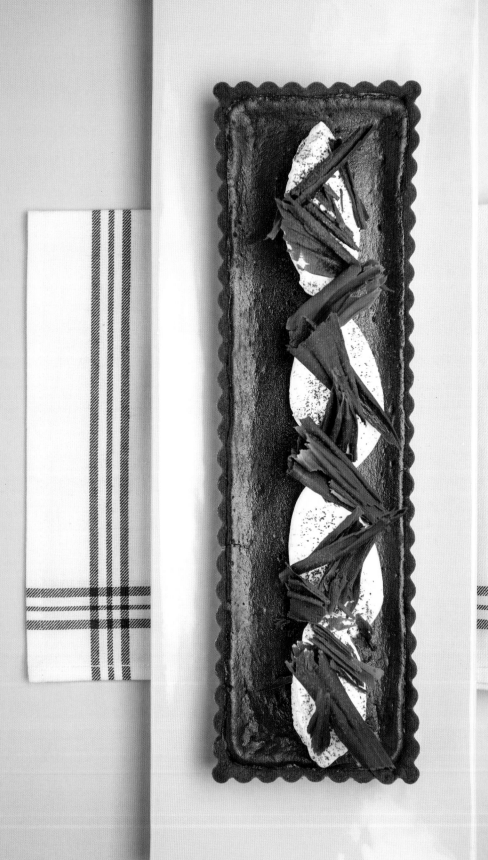

Belgian Chocolate Cheesecake

YIELD: 1 LONG (14-INCH × 4½-INCH × 1-INCH)
RECTANGULAR TART PAN / 8 SERVINGS

Eli's Belgian Chocolate Cheesecake is the richest, most intensely chocolate dessert I have ever tasted. When I was a little girl, my mother, Harriet, only made chocolate cheesecake for company. In fact, the recipe she used, which she'd cut out of a now-yellowed 1960s newspaper, called chocolate cheesecake "an unusual and elegant dessert you'll want to serve for a very special occasion."

We were so excited when we found out that the 2015 James Beard Awards were coming to Chicago, and even more so when we learned that Eli's had been invited to serve dessert to an incredible audience of James Beard Award winners and nominees at the event's welcome reception at Soho House. Diana and her team decided to create this recipe for the occasion, alongside a giant strawberry cheesecake.

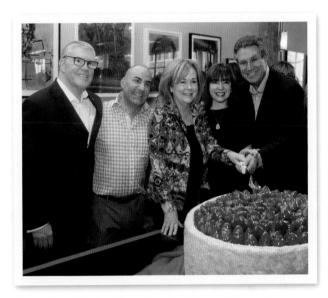

From left to right: Don Welsh, President, Choose Chicago; Sam Toia, President, Illinois Restaurant Association; Susan Ungaro, CEO, James Beard Foundation; and Maureen and Marc Schulman.
PHOTO BY LEIGH LOFTUS

Shopping List

FOR THE CHOCOLATE SHORTBREAD CRUST:

1½ sticks (12 tablespoons) cold unsalted butter

2/3 cup confectioners' sugar

1/2 teaspoon salt

1/4 teaspoon vanilla extract

1½ cups all-purpose flour

3 tablespoons cocoa powder

FOR THE BELGIAN CHOCOLATE GANACHE:

5 ounces Belgian bittersweet chocolate

1/3 cup heavy cream

RECIPE CONTINUES ON PAGE 154

BELGIAN CHOCOLATE CHEESECAKE (CONTINUED FROM PAGE 153)

FOR THE BELGIAN CHOCOLATE BATTER:

1 (8-ounce) package cream cheese, room temperature

⅓ cup granulated sugar

1 tablespoon cocoa powder

2 large whole eggs, room temperature

½ teaspoon vanilla extract

1. Prepare the Chocolate Shortbread Crust (see recipe on p. 113). Follow the recipe as directed. Roll out the dough in a rectangular shape to ¼-inch thick. Carefully lay the dough over the tart pan and gently press the dough into the sides and onto the bottom of the pan. Use a paring knife to cut off any excess dough.

2. Prepare the Belgian Chocolate Ganache and then the Belgian Chocolate batter (see recipes on pp. 83 and 82, respectively). Follow the recipes as directed.

3. Preheat the oven to 280°F. Pour the Belgian Chocolate batter into the prepared tart pan. Using an offset spatula, smooth down the batter until it is level.

4. Set the tart pan on a baking sheet and place the baking sheet in the center of the oven, directly on the middle shelf. Bake for 25 minutes, until the cake is slightly firm to the touch, jiggles in the center, and is lightly souffléd on the sides. Remove from the oven and set aside to cool to room temperature, about 1 hour.

5. Refrigerate for 4 hours or overnight to completely set before serving.

6. Transfer to the freezer for 2 to 3 hours before slicing.

7. Slice the tart with a thin, nonserrated knife that is dipped in hot water and wiped dry after each slice. Serve immediately or store in the freezer well wrapped for up to 3 months.

ELI'S TRADE SECRET *Always make sure the ganache is warm (about 110°F) when adding it to the batter; otherwise, it will not incorporate well.*

Caramel Pecan Pie Cheesecake Tart

YIELD: 1 (9-INCH) FLUTED TART PAN / 12 SERVINGS

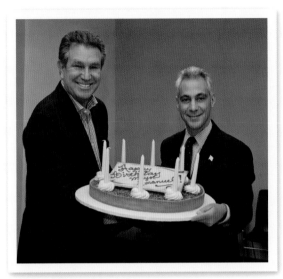

Marc presents Chicago Mayor Rahm Emanuel with a birthday pecan pie cheesecake

Chicago Mayor Rahm Emanuel has been a great fan and customer of Eli's Cheesecake since his 1993 election to the US Congress from the 5th District, which includes Eli's Cheesecake World. He began sending Eli's cheesecakes as a recruiting tool for potential candidates. Leading up to the 2006 congressional election, Emanuel sent out 70 Eli's cheesecakes to Democratic candidates, and the Democrats took over Congress for the first time in 12 years. It has been cited in numerous articles that Emanuel was known for treating his donors well by sending Eli's Cheesecake, but in the case of one pollster who upset him, he sent a 2½-foot-long dead fish instead. Marc quipped, "Eli's Cheesecake is the flip side to the dead fish." "All of Emanuel's cheesecakes always come with the same note," said Pete Giangreco, Emanuel's campaign spokesman: "Thank you, and enjoy one of Chicago's best. —Rahm." Of course the Mayor likes cheesecake, but his favorite dessert is pecan pie. One year for his birthday we made him a giant pecan pie cheesecake—a lot of pecan pie with a thin cheesecake layer at the bottom.

Shopping List

FOR THE CHOCOLATE SHORTBREAD CRUST:

1½ sticks (12 tablespoons) cold unsalted butter

2/3 cup confectioners' sugar

1/2 teaspoon salt

1/4 teaspoon vanilla extract

1½ cups all-purpose flour

3 tablespoons cocoa powder

FOR THE BELGIAN CHOCOLATE GANACHE:

5 ounces Belgian bittersweet chocolate

1/3 cup heavy cream

RECIPE CONTINUES ON PAGE 156

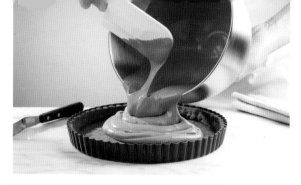

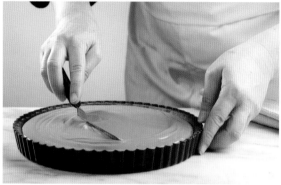

CARAMEL PECAN PIE CHEESECAKE TART

(CONTINUED FROM PAGE 155)

FOR THE BELGIAN CHOCOLATE BATTER:

- 1 (8-ounce) package cream cheese, room temperature
- 1/3 cup granulated sugar
- 1 tablespoon cocoa powder
- 2 large whole eggs, room temperature
- 1/2 teaspoon vanilla extract

FOR THE GARNISH:

- 6 ounces pecans, halved

FOR THE SALTED CARAMEL:

- 1 tablespoon corn syrup
- 2 tablespoons water
- 1/4 teaspoon salt
- 1 cup granulated sugar
- 3/4 cup heavy cream, warmed to at least 100°F

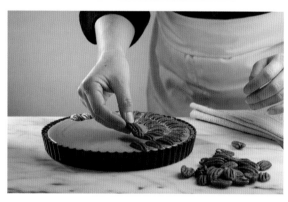

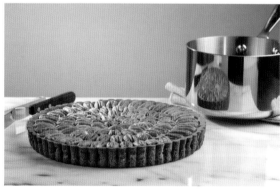

1. Prepare the Chocolate Shortbread Crust (see recipe on p. 113). Follow the recipe as directed. Roll out the dough in a circular shape to ¼-inch thick. Carefully lay the dough over the fluted tart pan and gently press the dough into the sides and onto the bottom of the pan. Use a paring knife to cut off any excess dough.

2. Prepare the Belgian Chocolate Ganache and then the Belgian Chocolate batter (see recipes on pp. 83 and 82, respectively). Follow the recipes as directed.

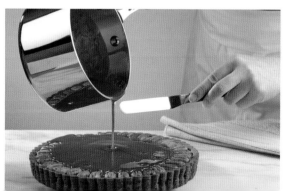

3. Preheat the oven to 300°F. Pour the Belgian Chocolate batter into the prepared tart pan. Using an offset spatula, smooth down the batter until it is level. Carefully arrange the pecan halves starting on the outside edge and working toward the center in concentric circles.

4. Set the tart pan in a baking sheet and place the baking sheet in the center of the oven, directly on the middle shelf. Bake for 15 to 20 minutes, until the cake jiggles very slightly (this is a shallow cake, so it shouldn't jiggle much). Remove from the oven and set aside to cool to room temperature, about 1 hour.

5. Prepare the Salted Caramel (see recipe on p. 128). Set aside to cool to 100°F.

6. Pour the Salted Caramel on the center of the cake. Using the back of a wooden spoon or a silicone offset spatula, spread the caramel evenly over the top of the cake, being careful not to spread over the cake's edge. Work quickly! As caramel cools, it begins to harden.

7. Refrigerate for 4 hours or overnight to completely set before serving.

8. Transfer to the freezer for 2 to 3 hours before slicing.

9. Slice the tart with a thin, nonserrated knife that is dipped in hot water and wiped dry after each slice. Serve immediately or store in the freezer well wrapped for up to 3 months.

ELI'S TRADE SECRET *Go with the flow...pour the hot caramel over a room-temperature cake to ensure that the caramel evenly spreads over the pecans.*

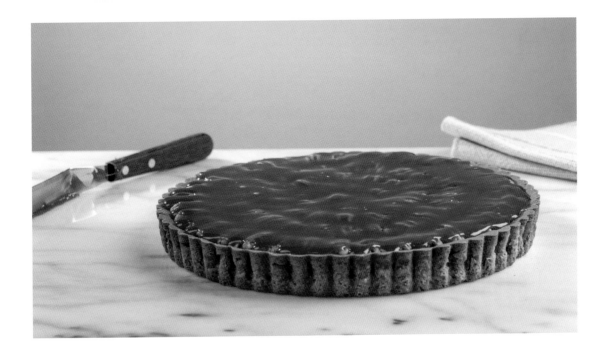

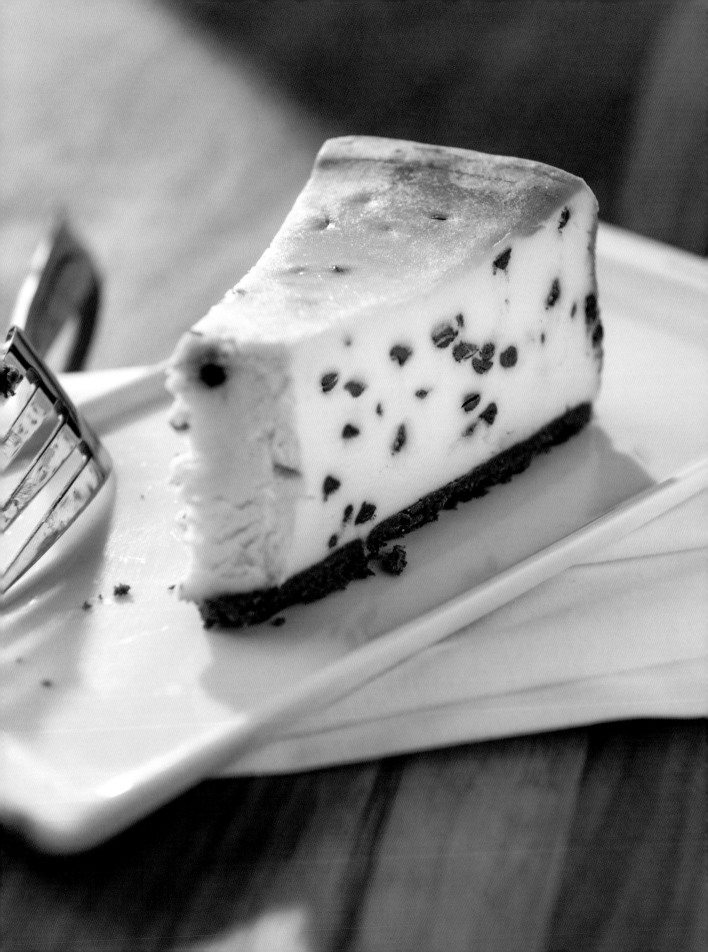

Chocolate Chip Cheesecake

YIELD: 1 (9-INCH) SPRINGFORM CHEESECAKE PAN / 12 SERVINGS

Chocolate chip was one of Eli's four originals, and it might just be the best flavor of all time. The small semi-sweet chocolate chips are a perfect foil for the tartness of the Original Plain batter. Jolene Worthington figured out that mini chips work much better than regular size chips, because they don't sink to the bottom. Before mini chips were readily available, we used to chop big blocks of chocolate into the exact sizes we needed.

We also make a cheesecake with a toffee candy bar. We wanted a certain size piece of toffee bar for baking, but no vendors provided that particular size. Around the same time, we noticed Ben and Jerry's ice cream had a flavor that contained just the size toffee piece we were looking for—so we called to see where they got them.

When Marc asked Jerry about it, he told him, "We drop the box of toffee off the roof of the barn." Sadly, Eli's doesn't have a barn.

Shopping List

FOR THE CHOCOLATE SHORTBREAD CRUST:

¾ stick (6 tablespoons) cold unsalted butter

⅓ cup confectioners' sugar

¼ teaspoon salt

⅛ teaspoon vanilla extract

¾ cup all-purpose flour

1½ tablespoons cocoa powder

FOR THE CHOCOLATE CHIP BATTER:

4 (8-ounce) packages cream cheese, room temperature

1 cup granulated sugar

¼ cup cake flour

¼ teaspoon salt

2 large whole eggs, room temperature

1 large egg yolk, room temperature

¾ cup sour cream, room temperature

½ teaspoon vanilla extract

1½ cups + 1 tablespoon miniature bittersweet chocolate chips

FOR THE GARNISH:

1 tablespoon chocolate chips (optional; see Trade Secret box)

RECIPE CONTINUES ON PAGE 160

CHOCOLATE CHIP CHEESECAKE (CONTINUED FROM PAGE 159)

1. Prepare ½ of the Chocolate Shortbread Crust recipe (see p. 113). Follow the recipe as directed. Roll out the dough in a circular shape to ¼-inch thick. Cut out 1 9-inch disc of dough and carefully place it in the bottom of a greased 9-inch springform pan.

2. Prepare the Chocolate Chip batter (see recipe on p. 84). Follow the recipe as directed.

3. Preheat the oven to 375°F. Generously grease and flour the springform pan (see Trade Secret on p. 76). Fill the springform pan with the Chocolate Chip batter. Using an offset spatula, smooth down the batter.

4. Place the filled springform pan in the center of the oven, directly on the middle shelf. Bake for 15 minutes, then rotate the cake 180 degrees to ensure even browning. (All ovens bake differently, so be alert for hot spots in your own oven.)

5. Bake for 15 minutes more, and again rotate the cake 180 degrees. The cake should be starting to soufflé and should be light in color. Continue to bake for 10 minutes more, for a total of 40 minutes at 375°F.

6. Reduce the oven temperature to 250°F and leave the oven door slightly ajar. The cakes should be golden brown and lightly souffléd on the sides. Leave the cake in the oven for 10 minutes more. (This step and the two that follow allow the cakes to cool to room temperature gently, preventing cracking.) Give the cake a gentle shake; it is done if the center of the cake jiggles and the surface of the cake is slightly firm. Turn the oven off and open the oven door wide. Leave the cake in the oven for 10 minutes more. Remove from the oven and set aside to cool to room temperature, about 1 hour.

7. Loosen the cheesecake from the springform pan by sliding an offset spatula around the inside ring. Remove the springform pan from the cake and transfer to a plate. Refrigerate for at least 8 hours or overnight before serving.

8. Transfer to the freezer for 2 to 3 hours before slicing.

9. Slice the cake with a thin, nonserrated knife that is dipped in hot water and wiped dry after each slice. Serve immediately or store in the freezer well wrapped for up to 3 months.

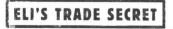

For a beautiful chocolate chip top, sprinkle an additional 1 tablespoon of chocolate chips over the top of the cake batter before baking.

Cinnamon Rum Raisin Cheesecake

YIELD: 1 (8-INCH OR 9-INCH) SPRINGFORM CHEESECAKE PAN OR 2 (6-INCH) SPRINGFORM
CHEESECAKE PANS

Back in the 1950s, Eli was a big fan of Little Jack's Restaurant, located at Madison and Kedzie. He loved their Cinnamon Raisin Cheesecake, which is why Cinnamon Raisin was one of his first four flavors. The first Eli's version used cottage cheese; he later switched to cream cheese and never looked back.

Eli's was recently asked to make a wedding cake for close family friends Jessica Farinella and Danny Flesh. While Jessie loves cheesecake, Danny only likes coffee cake. Eli's pastry chef extraordinaire Laurel Boger came up with a solution both could be happy with: She layered an all-butter yellow cake with a cinnamon–raisin cheesecake and coated the whole thing with old-fashioned buttercream frosting, creating the word's fanciest "coffee cake."

Eli's handwritten recipe.

RECIPE CONTINUES ON PAGE 163

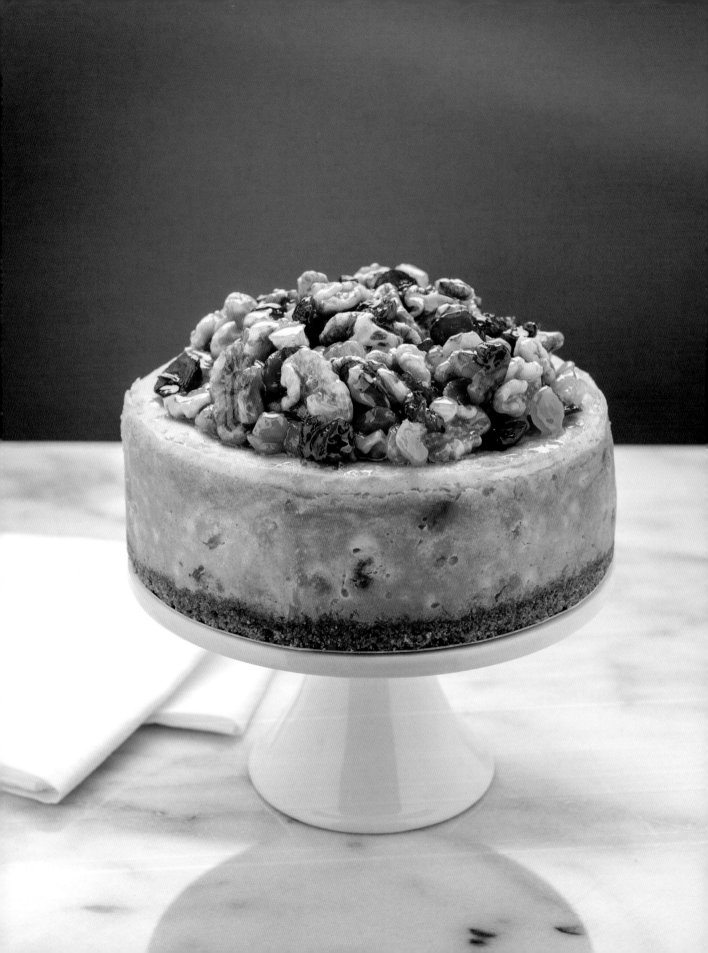

CINNAMON RUM RAISIN CHEESECAKE (CONTINUED FROM PAGE 161)

Shopping List

FOR THE GRAHAM CRUMB CRUST:

2 cups (16 ounces) finely ground graham cracker crumbs

¼ cup light brown sugar, firmly packed

¼ cup unsalted butter, melted

1 large egg white

FOR THE CANDIED WALNUTS:

1 cup water

1 cup granulated sugar

12 ounces walnuts

FOR THE PLUMPED RAISINS (2 RECIPES REQUIRED, DIVIDED):

2 cups golden raisins

2 cups boiling water

½ cup dark rum

¼ cup unsalted butter

FOR THE CINNAMON RUM RAISIN BATTER:

4 (8-ounce) packages cream cheese, room temperature

1 cup granulated sugar

¼ cup cake flour

½ teaspoon ground cinnamon

¼ teaspoon salt

2 large whole eggs, room temperature

1 large egg yolk, room temperature

¾ cup sour cream, room temperature

1 teaspoon vanilla extract

FOR THE GARNISH:

¼ cup honey

RECIPE CONTINUES ON PAGE 164

CINNAMON RUM RAISIN CHEESECAKE (CONTINUED FROM PAGE 163)

1. Prepare the Graham Crumb Crust (see recipe on p. 117) in 1 (8- or 9-inch) springform pan or two 6-inch springform pans. Follow the recipe as directed.

2. Prepare the Candied Walnuts (see recipe on p. 124) and 2 recipes of the Plumped Raisins (see recipe on p. 87). Follow the recipes as directed and set aside until ready for use.

3. Prepare the Cinnamon Rum Raisin batter (see recipe on p. 87). Follow the recipe as directed.

4. Preheat the oven to 300°F. Generously grease and flour the springform pan(s) (see Trade Secret on p. 76). Fill the springform pan(s) with the Cinnamon Rum Raisin batter. Using an offset spatula, smooth down the batter until it is level.

5. Place the filled springform pan(s) in the center of the oven, directly on the middle shelf. Bake for 45 to 50 minutes. The cake(s) should be golden brown and lightly souffléd on the sides. Give the cake(s) a gentle shake. The baking time is complete if the center of the cake(s) jiggles and the surface of the cake(s) is slightly firm. Remove from the oven and set aside to cool to room temperature, about 1 hour.

6. Refrigerate for at least 1 hour before removing the cake(s) from the pan(s).

7. Loosen the cheesecake from the springform pan by sliding an offset spatula around the inside ring. Remove the springform pan from the cake and transfer to a serving plate. Refrigerate 8 hours or overnight before decorating.

8. Decorate the cake by combining the ¼ cup honey with the Candied Walnuts and the reserved Plumped Raisins. Stir until well combined. Pour the mixture on top of the cheesecake.

9. Transfer to the freezer for 2 to 3 hours before slicing.

10. Slice the cake with a thin, nonserrated knife that is dipped in hot water and wiped dry after each slice. Serve immediately or store in the freezer well wrapped for up to 3 months.

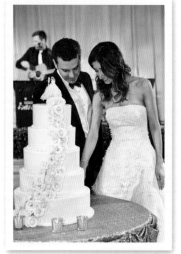

The Farinella-Flesh Cinnamon Rum Raisin wedding cake.
PHOTO BY KINGEN SMITH

Crème Fraîche No-Bake Cheesecake with Blackberries

YIELD: 8 (4-OUNCE) INDIVIDUAL SERVINGS

We decided to include a recipe for no-bake cheesecake because we wanted to cover every type of cheese-cake for this, our complete guide to America's favorite dessert. Refrigerated no-bake cheesecakes have been popular since the 1930s, when most homes had their own electric refrigerators. It's especially great for college dorms, where students usually don't have access to an oven. Believe it or not, dorm-room cheesecake is still a thing.

Shopping List

FOR THE ALMOND STREUSEL:

- ½ cup all-purpose flour
- ¾ cup granulated sugar
- 5 tablespoons cold unsalted butter
- ¼ teaspoon salt
- ¾ cup slivered almonds

FOR THE CRÈME FRAÎCHE NO-BAKE BATTER:

- 2 (8-ounce) packages cream cheese, room temperature
- ⅔ cup granulated sugar, divided
- ¾ cup crème fraîche
- 1 cup heavy cream
- 2 large egg yolks, room temperature
- 1 teaspoon vanilla extract
- 1 teaspoon unflavored gelatin powder
- 2 teaspoons cold water
- 2 cups water

FOR THE GARNISH:

- 2 cups Blackberry Compote (see recipe on p. 125)
- 1 tablespoon lemon zest (optional)

RECIPE CONTINUES ON PAGE 166

CRÈME FRAÎCHE NO-BAKE CHEESECAKE WITH BLACKBERRIES *(CONTINUED FROM PAGE 165)*

1. Prepare the Almond Streusel recipe (see p. 114). Follow the recipe as directed. Divide the streusel evenly into the bottoms of 8 (10-ounce) tumbler glasses arranged on a baking sheet.

2. Prepare the Crème Fraîche No-Bake batter (see recipe on p. 88). Follow the recipe as directed. While the batter is still fresh and has not yet firmed up, divide it evenly into each of the tumbler glasses. Pour slowly to ensure that the streusel is not displaced. (Use a pitcher with a pouring spout or a pastry bag to ensure a clean pour.) Refrigerate for 4 hours or overnight.

3. Just prior to serving, top the individual servings with the Blackberry Compote and the lemon zest, if using. Serve cold.

ELI'S TRADE SECRET *Ready Set Pour: Transfer the batter to the glasses immediately in order to prevent the gelatin from setting up too quickly.*

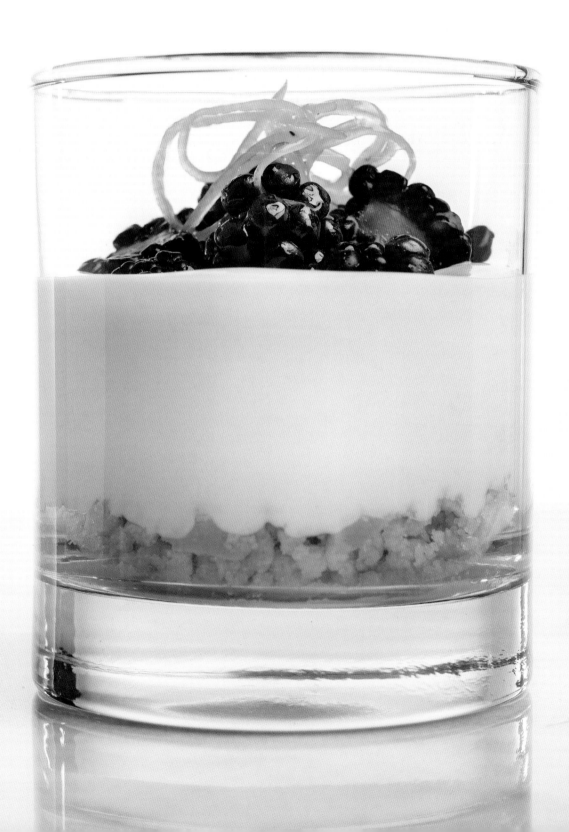

Eggnog Brûlée Cheesecake with Graham Crumb Crust

YIELD: 8 INDIVIDUAL (3-INCH) SPRINGFORM CHEESECAKE PANS / 8 SERVINGS

Nothing says "happy holidays" more than a gleaming punch bowl filled with eggnog. Come to think of it, eggnog is like liquid cheesecake—made with eggs, sugar, and cream, it's rich, sweet, thick, and creamy. Imagine how good eggnog could be if it were in a rum-spiked cheesecake on a crisp graham crumb crust!

Shopping List

FOR THE GRAHAM CRUMB CRUST:

2 cups (16 ounces) finely ground graham cracker crumbs

¼ cup light brown sugar, firmly packed

¼ cup unsalted butter, melted

1 large egg white

1 teaspoon nutmeg or cinnamon, depending on preference

FOR THE EGGNOG BATTER:

3 (8-ounce) packages cream cheese, room temperature

1 cup + 8 tablespoons granulated sugar, divided

¼ cup cake flour

1 teaspoon ground nutmeg

4 large egg yolks, room temperature

1 cup eggnog, divided, room temperature

½ teaspoon vanilla extract

2 tablespoons dark rum (optional)

1. Prepare the Graham Crumb Crust (see recipe on p. 117) in 8 individual (3-inch) springform pans. For a festive flair, add 1 teaspoon nutmeg or cinnamon to step 2 of the recipe. Press about ¼ cup of the mixture into each pan in step 6. Otherwise, follow the recipe as directed.

2. Prepare the Eggnog batter (see recipe on p. 90). Follow the recipe as directed.

3. Preheat the oven to 275°F. Generously grease and flour the springform pans (see Trade Secret on p. 76). Evenly space the pans on baking sheets and fill them with the Eggnog batter. Using an offset spatula, smooth down the batter until it is level in each pan.

4. Place the filled springform pans in the center of the oven. Bake for 20 to 25 minutes, until the cakes start to soufflé. Give the cakes a gentle shake. The baking time is complete if the center of the cakes jiggle slightly. Remove from the oven and set aside to cool to room temperature, about 1 hour.

5. Refrigerate for at least 1 hour before removing the cakes from the pans.

6. Loosen the cheesecake from the springform pans by sliding an offset spatula around the inside ring. Remove the springform pans from the cakes. Refrigerate 8 hours or overnight. Just before serving, place cheesecakes on a metal surface. Sprinkle the top of each with the remaining tablespoons of granulated sugar and torch until caramelized.

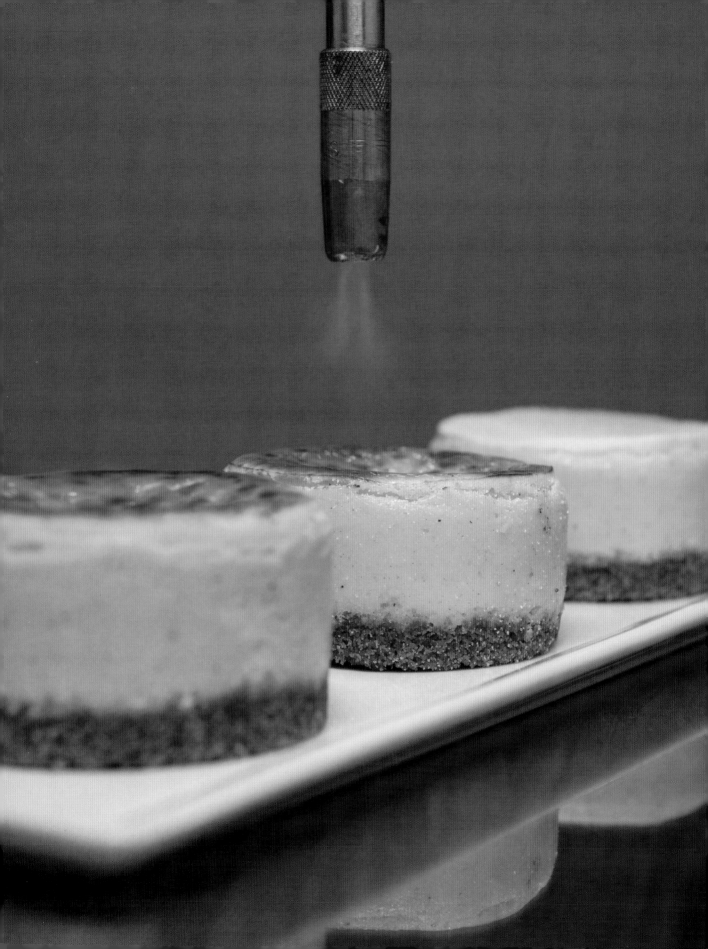

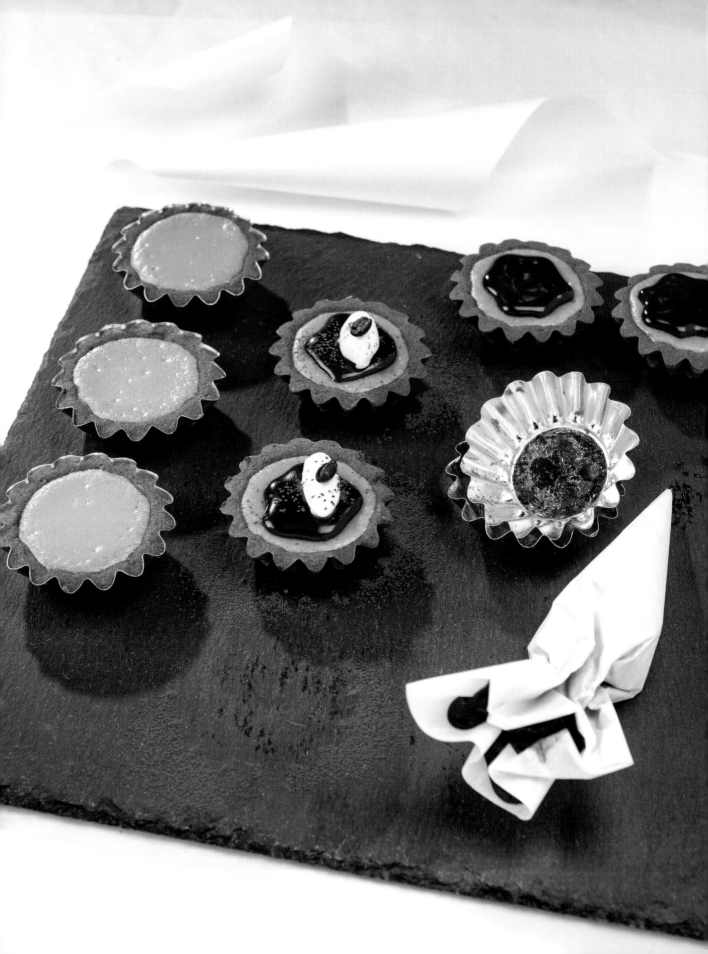

Espresso Cheesecake Tartlets

YIELD: 18 (2-INCH) TARTLET PANS / 18 SERVINGS

Hillary Rodham Clinton celebrated her 50th birthday in Chicago, and Eli's was there. We prepared a giant cheesecake consisting of layers of espresso and chocolate chip cheesecakes—her favorite flavors. Try these tartlets for great taste on a significantly smaller scale.

Shopping List

FOR THE CHOCOLATE SHORTBREAD CRUST:

1½ sticks (12 tablespoons) cold unsalted butter

2/3 cup confectioners' sugar

½ teaspoon salt

¼ teaspoon vanilla extract

1½ cups all-purpose flour

3 tablespoons cocoa powder

FOR THE ESPRESSO BATTER:

2 (8-ounce) packages cream cheese, room temperature

¾ cup granulated sugar

1 tablespoon cake flour

Pinch salt

1 large whole egg, room temperature

1 large egg yolk, room temperature

2 teaspoons instant coffee or espresso

2 teaspoons boiling water

¼ cup sour cream, room temperature

½ teaspoon vanilla extract

FOR THE BELGIAN CHOCOLATE GANACHE:

5 ounces Belgian bittersweet chocolate

1/3 cup heavy cream

FOR THE GARNISH:

½ cup crème fraîche

1 teaspoon cocoa powder

RECIPE CONTINUES ON PAGE 172

ESPRESSO CHEESECAKE TARTLETS (CONTINUED FROM PAGE 171)

1. Prepare the Chocolate Shortbread Crust (see recipe on p. 113). Place the 18 tartlet pans on a pair of baking sheets. Roll out the dough in a circular shape to ¼-inch thick. Using a 3-inch round cookie cutter or drinking glass, cut out 18 3-inch discs of dough. Using your fingers, press the discs into the tartlet pans, making sure to evenly spread the dough on the bottom and up the sides of each pan. Use a paring knife to trim away any excess dough. Follow the recipe through Step 7, and then transfer the baking sheets to the oven and bake for 8 minutes. *Note: Tartlet crusts bake quickly—set your timer to be sure you don't overbake the crusts.* Remove from the oven and set aside to cool.

2. Prepare the Espresso batter (see recipe on p. 93). Follow the recipe as directed.

3. Preheat the oven to 250°F. Using a piping bag, pour the Espresso batter into the prepared tartlet pans.

4. Transfer the baking sheets to the oven and bake for 10 to 12 minutes. Watch the tartlets carefully throughout the baking time, as you must take care not to overbake them. Remove from the oven and set aside to cool to room temperature, about 1 hour.

5. Prepare the Belgian Chocolate Ganache (see recipe on p. 83). Follow the recipe as directed and set aside while still warm, but not hot.

6. Using a piping bag, decorate each tartlet with 1 tablespoon of the Belgian Chocolate Ganache. Set aside to cool completely for 1 hour.

7. Refrigerate for 1 hour to completely set before garnishing.

8. Garnish each tartlet with a dollop of the crème fraîche and a light dusting of the cocoa powder. Serve.

ELI'S TRADE SECRET *In order to achieve the best espresso coffee flavor, use freeze-dried instant coffee and never brewed coffee.*

Fresh Cheese Cheesecake Tarts with Huckleberries

YIELD: 12 INDIVIDUAL (3-INCH) TART PANS / 12 SERVINGS

It is a well-known fact that President Barack Obama loves huckleberry pie. The first one we ever made for him was served on a flight aboard Air Force One from Chicago to Washington, to celebrate his 50th birthday with those on board. The second time Eli's made a huckleberry dessert for President Obama was on a visit to Chicago for a fundraiser at the home of Grace Tsao-Wu and Craig Freedman. Tara Lane, a coauthor of this book, baked pies for the Obamas from the time the President was a senator and lived in Chicago until the family moved to Washington, DC. This time, Tara made deconstructed individual cheesecakes with a delicious fresh huckleberry topping, served warm. Once again, the President saved his dessert to have on the way back to the White House.

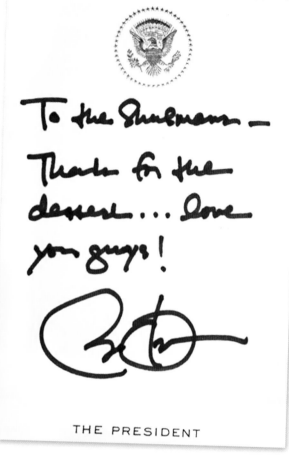

A thank-you note from President Obama regarding the huckleberry cheesecake.

Shopping List

FOR THE HUCKLEBERRY COMPOTE:

- 2½ cups frozen huckleberries
- ¼ cup granulated sugar
- 1 tablespoon fresh lemon juice
- Zest of 1 lemon

FOR THE SHORTBREAD CRUST:

- 1½ sticks (12 tablespoons) cold unsalted butter
- ½ cup confectioners' sugar
- ½ teaspoon salt
- ¼ teaspoon vanilla extract
- 1½ cups all-purpose flour

RECIPE CONTINUES ON PAGE 175

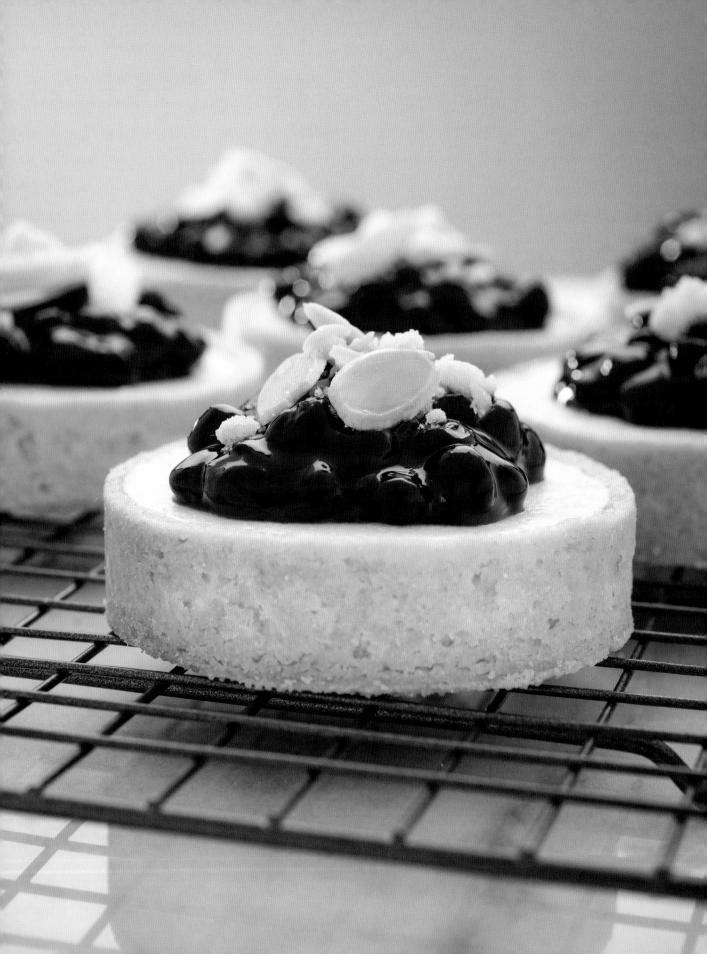

FRESH CHEESE CHEESECAKE TARTS WITH HUCKLEBERRIES *(CONTINUED FROM PAGE 173)*

FOR THE ALMOND STREUSEL:

½ cup all-purpose flour

¾ cup granulated sugar

5 tablespoons cold unsalted butter

¼ teaspoon salt

¾ cup slivered almonds

FOR THE FRESH CHEESE BATTER:

½ cup ricotta cheese, room temperature

6 ounces goat cheese, room temperature

½ cup mascarpone cheese, room temperature

12 ounces cream cheese, room temperature

½ cup sour cream, room temperature

¾ cup granulated sugar, divided

1 tablespoon cake flour

1 teaspoon lemon zest

3 large egg whites, room temperature

4 large egg yolks, room temperature

1. Prepare the Huckleberry Compote (see recipe on p. 126). Follow the recipe as directed and store in the refrigerator until ready for use.

2. Preheat the oven to 325°F.

3. Prepare the Shortbread Crust (see recipe on p. 110). Follow the recipe as directed through Step 4. Place the 12 tartlet pans on a pair of baking sheets. Roll out the dough in a circular shape to ¼-inch thick. Using a 4-inch round cookie cutter or drinking glass, cut out 12 4-inch discs of dough. Using your fingers, press the discs into the tart pans, making sure to evenly spread the dough on the bottom and up the sides of each pan. Use a paring knife to trim away any excess dough. Transfer the baking sheets to the oven and bake for 12 minutes, until golden brown. *Note: Tart crusts bake quickly—set your timer to be sure you don't overbake the crusts.* Remove from the oven and set aside to cool.

4. Prepare the Almond Streusel recipe (see p. 114). Follow the recipe as directed. Set aside until ready for use.

RECIPE CONTINUES ON PAGE 176

FRESH CHEESE CHEESECAKE TARTS WITH
HUCKLEBERRIES *(CONTINUED FROM PAGE 175)*

5. Prepare the Fresh Cheese batter (see recipe on pp. 95). Follow the recipe as directed.

6. Lower the oven temperature to 275°F. Using a piping bag, pour the Fresh Cheese batter into the prepared tart shells. Fill each shell to the top and gently tap the side of the baking pan to smooth or level out the filling. *Note: This is a very light and fragile batter, so be careful not to overwork it.*

7. Transfer the baking sheets to the oven and bake for 12 to 15 minutes, until the centers are slightly firm to the touch. Watch the tarts carefully throughout the baking time, as you must take care not to overbake them. Remove from the oven and set aside to cool to room temperature, about 1 hour.

8. Refrigerate for 1 hour to completely set before garnishing.

9. Garnish each tart with a few spoonfuls of the Huckleberry Compote and sprinkle the Almond Streusel over the berries. Serve.

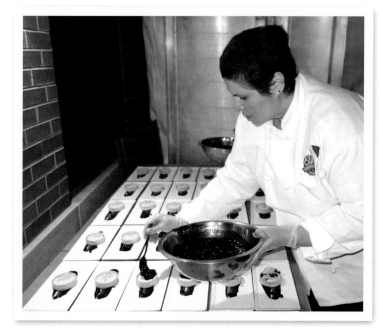

Juanita plating up the Huckleberry Cheesecake for the President on-site.

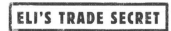 Our favorite locally sourced goat cheese comes from Capriole Farms in Greenville, Indiana.

Honey Almond Pistachio Ricotta Cheesecake

YIELD: 1 (9-INCH) SPRINGFORM CHEESECAKE PAN / 12 SERVINGS

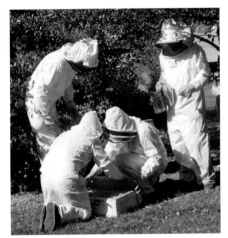 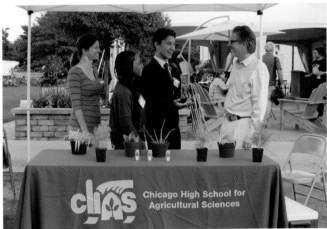

FROM LEFT: *CHSAS students collect honey from the school's hives; Jeff Anderson talks to CHSAS students during the school's summer program at Eli's.*

When Eli's was looking for a source of premium honey for our Mediterranean Honey Cheesecake and other desserts with a taste of honey, we didn't have to look very far. For over 25 years now, Eli's has partnered with the Chicago High School for Agricultural Sciences (CHSAS), one of the few high schools in the country located on a working farm.

On its 40-acre farm, CHSAS maintains 22 beehives. Students are involved in the entire process, from harvesting and producing to packaging the honey. Proceeds from honey sales go toward college scholarships for deserving high school seniors. In addition, The Eli's Cheesecake Company provides four University of Illinois scholarships annually to students interested in pursuing careers in food.

Shopping List

FOR THE TOASTED ALMOND CRUST:

1 cup whole skinned almonds, toasted

2 tablespoons granulated sugar

½ teaspoon salt

1 tablespoon unsalted butter, melted

RECIPE CONTINUES ON PAGE 179

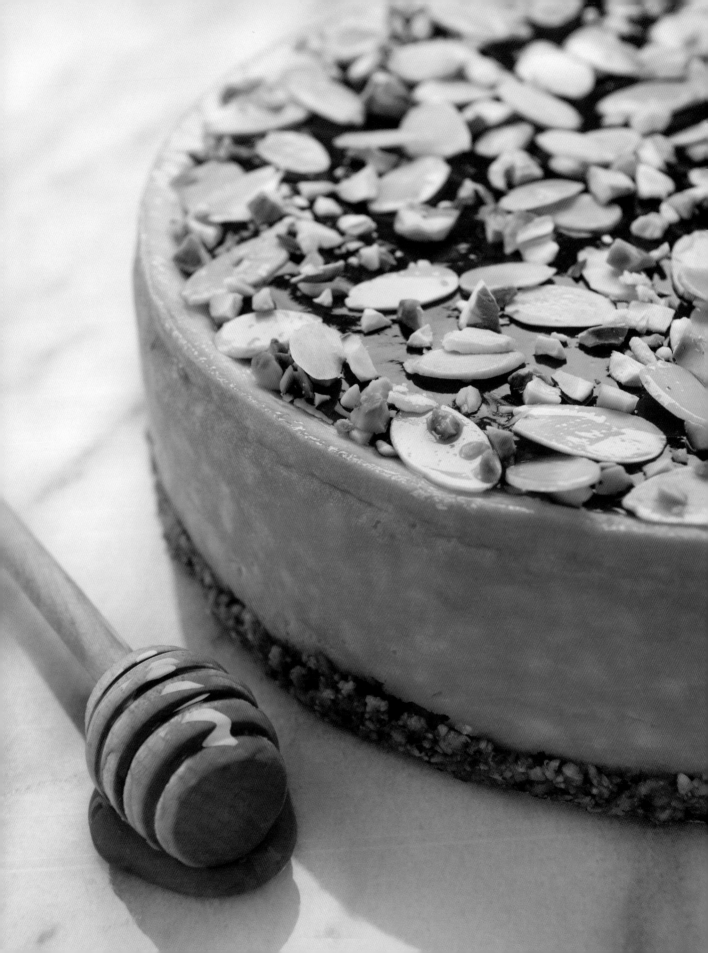

HONEY ALMOND PISTACHIO RICOTTA CHEESECAKE

(CONTINUED FROM PAGE 177)

FOR THE HONEY RICOTTA BATTER:

15 ounces ricotta cheese, room temperature

2 (8-ounce) packages cream cheese, room temperature

½ cup granulated sugar

¼ teaspoon salt

2 tablespoons cake flour

¼ cup honey

½ teaspoon vanilla extract

2 large whole eggs, room temperature

½ cup sour cream, room temperature

FOR THE HONEY CARAMEL:

½ cup honey

⅓ cup granulated sugar

½ tablespoon molasses

¼ teaspoon salt

¼ cup heavy cream

FOR THE GARNISH:

¼ cup slivered almonds, toasted

¼ cup chopped pistachios

1. Prepare the Toasted Almond Crust (see recipe on p. 118) in a 9-inch springform pan. Follow the recipe as directed.

2. Prepare the Honey Ricotta batter (see recipe on p. 99). Follow the recipe as directed.

3. Preheat the oven to 300°F. Generously grease and flour the springform pan (see Trade Secret on p. 76). Fill the springform pan with the Honey Ricotta batter.

4. Place the filled springform pan in the center of the oven, directly on the middle shelf. Bake for 45 to 50 minutes, until the cake is slightly firm to the touch, jiggles in the center, and is lightly souf-fléd on the sides. Remove from the oven and set aside to cool to room temperature, about 1 hour.

RECIPE CONTINUES ON PAGE 180

HONEY ALMOND PISTACHIO RICOTTA CHEESECAKE

(CONTINUED FROM PAGE 179)

5. Loosen the cheesecake from the springform pan by sliding an offset spatula around the inside ring. Remove the springform pan from the cake and transfer to a plate. Refrigerate for at least 8 hours or overnight before serving.

6. Prepare the Honey Caramel (see recipe on p. 128). Set aside while still warm, but not hot.

7. Pour the Honey Caramel on the center of the room-temperature cake. Using the back of a wooden spoon or a silicone offset spatula, spread the caramel evenly over the top of the cake, being careful not to spread over the cake's edge. Sprinkle the almonds and pistachios on the top of the cake. Work quickly! As caramel cools, it begins to harden.

8. Refrigerate for 4 hours or overnight to completely set before serving.

9. Transfer to the freezer for 2 to 3 hours before slicing.

10. Slice the cake with a thin, nonserrated knife that is dipped in hot water and wiped dry after each slice. Serve immediately or store in the freezer well wrapped for up to 3 months.

ELI'S TRADE SECRET *Experiment with various brands and types of honey to create cakes with subtly different flavor profiles.*

Honey Ricotta Illinois Prairie Cheesecake with Candied Blood Oranges

YIELD: 1 (9-INCH) SPRINGFORM CHEESECAKE PAN / 12 SERVINGS

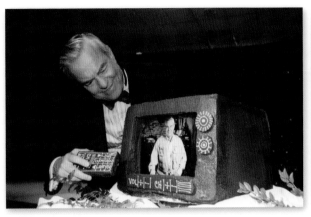 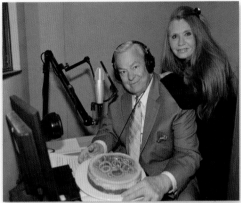

FROM LEFT: *Eli's created a TV cheesecake for Bill Kurtis when he was honored by the Museum of Broadcast Communications, 1999; Bill and Donna at the studio with the Honey Ricotta Illinois Prairie Cheesecake.*

Like Eli's Cheesecake, Bill Kurtis and Donna LaPietra are symbols of Chicago. Bill, the renowned television journalist, and Donna, Executive Producer of Kurtis Productions, are big Eli's Cheesecake fans. When we invited them to imagine a number-one-in-the-ratings cheesecake, they came up with Illinois Prairie Cheesecake, calling out their commitment to restoring native prairies.

Shopping List

FOR THE TOASTED OAT AND PECAN STREUSEL:

1 cup all-purpose flour

½ cup light brown sugar

5 tablespoons cold unsalted butter

½ teaspoon ground cinnamon

¼ teaspoon salt

¼ cup lightly toasted oats

¼ cup chopped pecans

FOR THE CANDIED BLOOD ORANGES:

3 blood oranges

1 cup water

1 cup granulated sugar

RECIPE CONTINUES ON PAGE 182

HONEY RICOTTA ILLINOIS PRAIRIE CHEESECAKE WITH CANDIED BLOOD ORANGES (CONTINUED FROM PAGE 181)

FOR THE HONEY RICOTTA BATTER:

15 ounces ricotta cheese, room temperature

2 (8-ounce) packages cream cheese, room temperature

½ cup granulated sugar

¼ teaspoon salt

2 tablespoons cake flour

¼ cup honey

½ teaspoon vanilla extract

2 large whole eggs, room temperature

½ cup sour cream, room temperature

> **ELI'S TRADE SECRET**
>
> *The longer the Candied Blood Oranges remain in the simple syrup, the more translucent and beautiful they become.*

1. Prepare the Toasted Oat and Pecan Streusel (see recipe variation on p. 115) in a 9-inch spring-form pan. Follow the recipe as directed through Step 4. Place the springform pan in the center of the oven, directly on the middle shelf. Bake for 15 minutes, until set. Watch the streusel through the bake time to ensure it is not overbaked. Remove from the oven and set aside to cool to room temperature, about 1 hour.

2. Prepare the the Candied Blood Oranges (see recipe on p. 123). Follow the recipe as directed and set aside until ready to use.

3. Prepare the Honey Ricotta batter (see recipe on p. 99). Follow the recipe as directed.

4. Preheat the oven to 300°F. Generously grease and flour the springform pan (see Trade Secret on p. 76). Fill the springform pan with the Honey Ricotta batter.

5. Place the filled springform pan in the center of the oven, directly on the middle shelf. Bake for 45 to 50 minutes, until the cake is slightly firm to the touch, jiggles in the center, and is lightly souf-fléd on the sides. Remove from the oven and set aside to cool to room temperature, about 1 hour.

6. Loosen the cheesecake from the springform pan by sliding an offset spatula around the inside ring. Remove the springform pan from the cake and transfer to a plate. Refrigerate for at least 1 hour or overnight before decorating.

7. Carefully place the Candied Blood Oranges on the top of the cake in a pattern of your choice.

8. Slice the cake with a thin, nonserrated knife that is dipped in hot water and wiped dry after each slice. Serve immediately or store in the freezer well wrapped for up to 3 months.

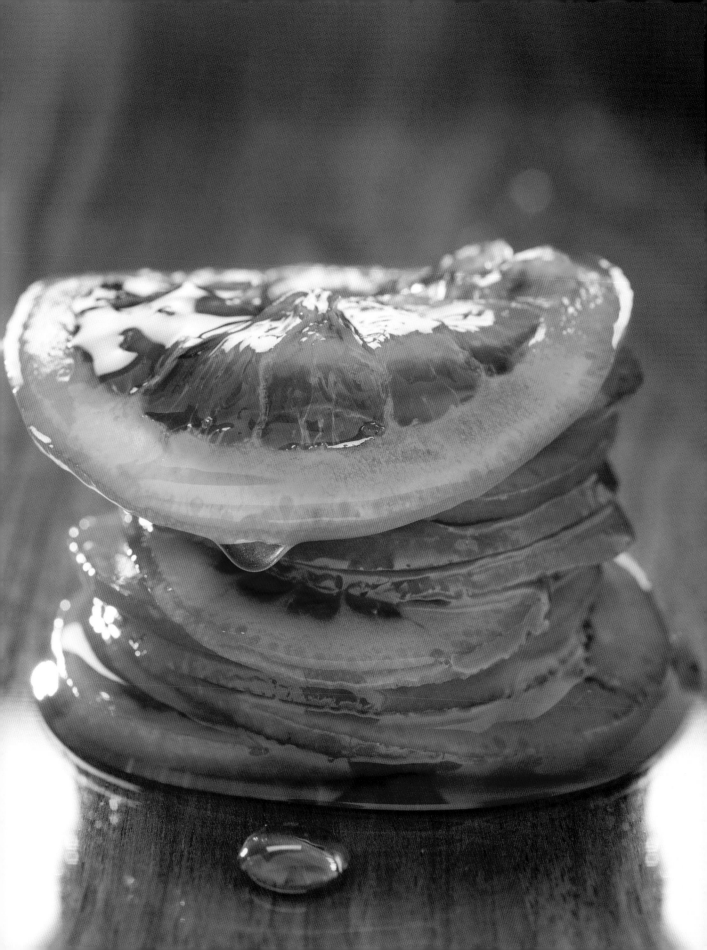

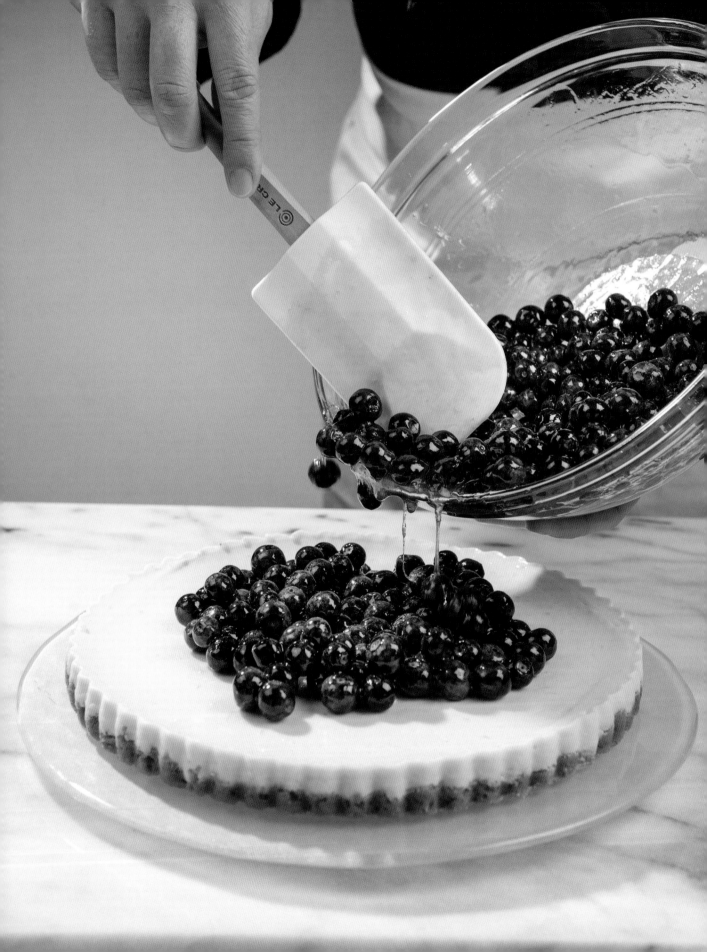

Lemon Cheesecake Tart with Blueberries

YIELD: 1 (9-INCH) FLUTED TART PAN / 12 SERVINGS

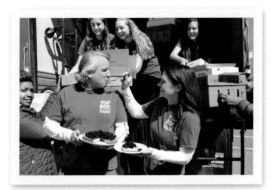

Chris and Sheila try their cheesecake during a Top Box delivery.

One of the many charity partners Eli's Cheesecake is proud to work with is Top Box Foods, a nonprofit hunger relief program founded by Chris Kennedy, son of the late Robert F. Kennedy, and Chris's wife, Sheila. By utilizing bulk purchasing power to get high-quality foods at a discount, Top Box is able to offer community residents the opportunity to purchase affordable fresh fruits, vegetables, and protein at monthly delivery locations throughout Chicago and Lake County. Eli's has donated cheesecake and desserts to Top Box since the organization's inception in 2012. When we asked Chris and Sheila to dream up their favorite cheesecake, they suggested Lemon Blueberry—a shout-out to the importance of the fresh fruit component in the Top Box deliveries.

Shopping List

FOR THE BLUEBERRY COMPOTE:

- 2 cups (15 ounces) fresh blueberries, rinsed, dried, and stems removed
- 8 ounces apricot jam
- 2 tablespoons water

FOR THE BROWN SUGAR STREUSEL:

- 1 cup all-purpose flour
- 1/2 cup light brown sugar
- 5 tablespoons cold unsalted butter
- 1/2 teaspoon ground cinnamon
- 1/4 teaspoon salt

FOR THE LEMON BATTER:

- 1 1/2 (8-ounce) packages cream cheese, room temperature
- 1 tablespoon lemon zest
- 1/2 cup granulated sugar, divided
- 1/2 teaspoon vanilla extract
- 2 large whole eggs, room temperature

RECIPE CONTINUES ON PAGE 186

LEMON CHEESECAKE TART WITH BLUEBERRIES

(CONTINUED FROM PAGE 185)

1. Prepare the Blueberry Compote (see recipe on p. 125). Follow the recipe as directed and store in the refrigerator until ready for use.

2. Prepare the Brown Sugar Streusel (see recipe on p. 115). Follow the recipe as directed.

3. Prepare the Lemon batter (see recipe on p. 100). Follow the recipe as directed.

4. Preheat the oven to 300°F. Fill the fluted tart pan with the Lemon batter.

5. Place the fluted tart pan in the center of the oven, directly on the middle shelf. Bake for 20 to 25 minutes, until the cake is slightly firm to the touch (this is a shallow cake, so it shouldn't jiggle much). Remove from the oven and set aside to cool to room temperature, about 1 hour.

6. Refrigerate for 4 hours or overnight to completely set before serving.

7. Before serving, pour the Blueberry Compote on the center of the cake. Using the back of a wooden spoon or a silicone offset spatula, spread the compote evenly over the top of the cake, being careful not to spread over the cake's edge.

8. Slice the tart with a thin, nonserrated knife that is dipped in hot water and wiped dry after each slice. Serve immediately.

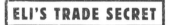 *You can use any berry at all to make a compote with the Quick Apricot Glaze.*

Pumpkin Cheesecake

YIELD: 1 (9-INCH) PIE PAN / 12 SERVINGS

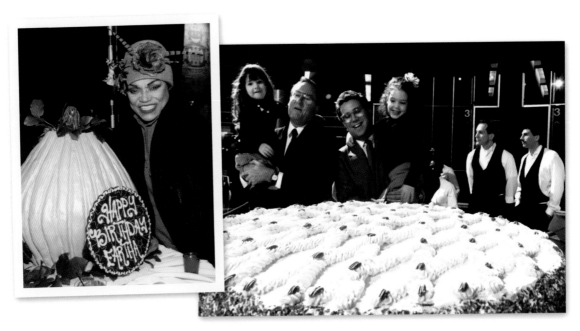

LEFT: *While in Chicago to portray the Fairy Godmother in Rodgers & Hammerstein's Cinderella, Eartha Kitt celebrated a birthday. So naturally, we made her a pumpkin cheesecake and presented it to her on stage.*

RIGHT: *Eli's baked up a giant pumpkin cheesecake for Thanksgiving and presented it in the beautiful lobby of the State of Illinois Building. In the photo, Governor Jim Thompson holds up Kori Schulman and Marc holds her sister Haley, showing off the scale of the cake.*

Come fall, America goes pumpkin crazy…pumpkin lattes, pumpkin ice cream, even pumpkin bagels! As far as desserts go, this delicious custardy pumpkin cheesecake can't be beat. Once, we baked a giant 1,000-pound version of this cake and served it to the public in the lobby of the State of Illinois Building.

Some Thanksgivings, I change things up by baking the batter in individual ramekins. After removing the ramekins from the refrigerator, just before serving, I sprinkle each one with sugar and torch for a crunchy brulée top.

Family-owned Stahlbush Island Farms in Oregon supplies our pumpkin purée, but canned pumpkin works well in this recipe. Be sure to buy canned pumpkin and not pumpkin pie filling…that's something different altogether.

RECIPE CONTINUES ON PAGE 189

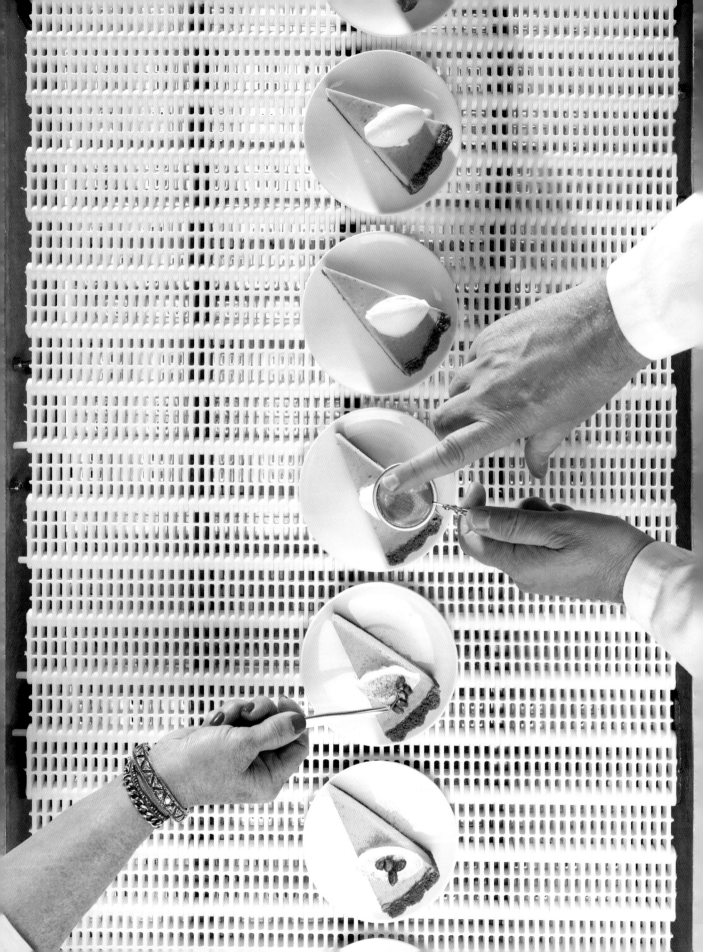

PUMPKIN CHEESECAKE (CONTINUED FROM PAGE 187)

Shopping List

FOR THE CINNAMON GRAHAM CRUMB CRUST:

2 cups (16 ounces) finely ground graham cracker crumbs

¼ cup light brown sugar, firmly packed

½ teaspoon ground cinnamon

¼ cup unsalted butter, melted

1 large egg white

FOR THE PUMPKIN BATTER:

3 (8-ounce) packages cream cheese, room temperature

1 cup granulated sugar

¼ cup cake flour

1 teaspoon pumpkin pie spice

¼ teaspoon ground nutmeg

½ teaspoon ground ginger

½ teaspoon salt

2 large whole eggs, room temperature

¾ cup canned pumpkin

⅓ cup sour cream, room temperature

1 teaspoon vanilla extract

ELI'S TRADE SECRET

For a different twist, substitute cooked sweet potatoes or cooked butternut squash for the canned pumpkin.

1. Prepare the Cinnamon Graham Crumb Crust (see recipe variation on p. 117) in a 9-inch pie pan. Follow the recipe as directed.

2. Prepare the Pumpkin batter (see recipe on p. 101). Follow the recipe as directed.

3. Preheat the oven to 280°F. Fill the fluted tart pan with the Pumpkin batter.

4. Place the fluted tart pan in the center of the oven, directly on the middle shelf. Bake for 35 to 40 minutes, until the cake is slightly firm to the touch (this is a shallow cake, so it shouldn't jiggle much). Remove from the oven and set aside to cool to room temperature, about 1 hour.

5. Refrigerate for 4 hours or overnight to completely set before serving.

6. Transfer to the freezer for 2 to 3 hours before slicing.

7. Slice the cake with a thin, nonserrated knife that is dipped in hot water and wiped dry after each slice. Serve immediately or store in the freezer well wrapped for up to 3 months.

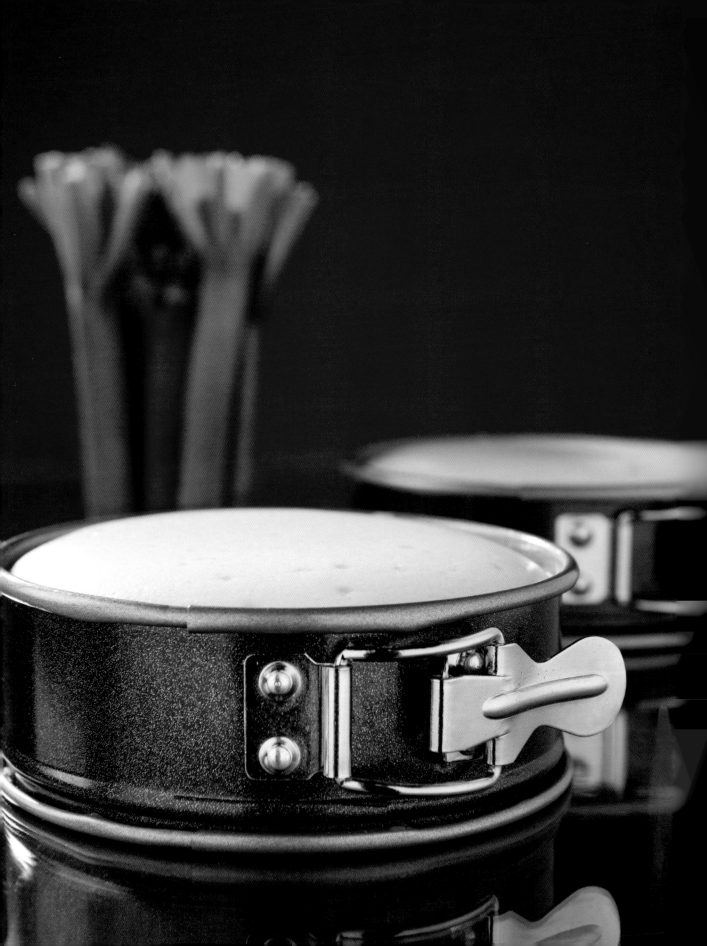

Sabayon Cheesecake with Rhubarb

YIELD: 6 INDIVIDUAL (4-INCH) SPRINGFORM CHEESECAKE PANS / 6 SERVINGS

If you've been waiting all winter for fresh fruit, you can count on rhubarb to be among the first yields of springtime. Our rhubarb comes to us from Stahlbush Island Farms, located in Oregon's lush Willamette Valley. Family owned since 1885, Stahlbush Island Farms is an environmentally friendly farm and food processor committed to sustainable agriculture.

FOR THE BROWN SUGAR STREUSEL:

1 cup all-purpose flour

½ cup light brown sugar

5 tablespoons cold unsalted butter

½ teaspoon ground cinnamon

¼ teaspoon salt

FOR THE RHUBARB COMPOTE:

2 cups (1½ pounds) ½-inch pieces fresh rhubarb

¾ cups granulated sugar

1 tablespoon fresh orange juice

FOR THE SABAYON BATTER:

2 cups water

5 large egg yolks, room temperature

4 (8-ounce) packages cream cheese, room temperature

1 cup granulated sugar, divided

3 tablespoons cake flour

2 large whole eggs, room temperature

¾ cup (6 ounces) sour cream, room temperature

1 teaspoon vanilla extract

1. Prepare the Brown Sugar Streusel (see recipe on p. 115). Follow the recipe as directed through Step 4. Measure ⅓ cup of the Brown Sugar Streusel into each of the springform pans and press down firmly. Place the 6 pans on a pair of baking sheets. Transfer the baking sheets to the oven and bake for 8 to 10 minutes until golden brown. Remove from the oven and set aside to cool.

2. Prepare the Rhubarb Compote (see recipe on p. 127). Follow the recipe as directed and store in the refrigerator until ready for use.

3. Prepare the Sabayon batter (see recipe on pp. 104). Follow the recipe as directed.

RECIPE CONTINUES ON PAGE 192

SABAYON CHEESECAKE WITH RHUBARB

(CONTINUED FROM PAGE 191)

4. Preheat the oven to 280°F. Generously grease and flour the springform pan (see Trade Secret on p. 76). Pour the Sabayon batter into the prepared springform pans. Using an offset spatula, smooth down the batter until it is level.

5. Place the baking sheets in the center of the oven, directly on the middle shelf. Bake for 30 minutes, until the cakes are slightly firm to the touch, jiggle in the center, and are lightly souffléd on the sides. Remove from the oven and set aside to cool to room temperature, about 1 hour.

6. Loosen the cheesecakes from the springform pans by sliding an offset spatula around the inside rings. Remove the springform pans from the cakes and transfer to plates. Refrigerate for at least 8 hours or overnight before serving.

7. Place the cheesecake in the freezer for 2 to 3 hours before slicing.

8. Slice the cake with a thin, nonserrated knife that is dipped in hot water and wiped dry after each slice. Serve immediately or store in the freezer well wrapped for up to 3 months.

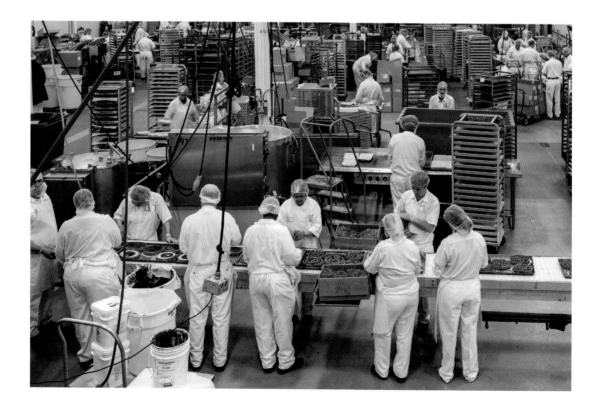

Salted Caramel Flan Cheesecake

YIELD: 1 (9-INCH) SPRINGFORM CHEESECAKE PAN / 12 SERVINGS

This is one of my favorite cheesecakes. I take it to every party I'm invited to as a hostess gift. It is sweet, salty, creamy, and crunchy all at the same time. Eli's Cheesecake originally started experimenting with nut crusts because our daughter Haley can't have flour, but she still loves cheesecake! It has become one of Eli's top sellers.

Shopping List

FOR THE TOASTED ALMOND CRUST:

1 cup whole skinned almonds, toasted

2 tablespoons granulated sugar

½ teaspoon salt

1 tablespoon unsalted butter, melted

FOR THE FLAN BATTER:

3 (8-ounce) packages cream cheese, room temperature

14 ounces sweetened condensed milk, divided

1 large whole egg, room temperature

5 large egg yolks, room temperature

1 teaspoon vanilla extract

FOR THE SALTED CARAMEL:

1 tablespoon corn syrup

2 tablespoons water

¼ teaspoon salt

1 cup granulated sugar

¾ cup heavy cream, warmed to at least 100°F

FOR THE GARNISH:

½ cup whole skinned almonds, toasted

Maldon sea salt crystals, to taste

RECIPE CONTINUES ON PAGE 194

SALTED CARAMEL FLAN CHEESECAKE *(CONTINUED FROM PAGE 193)*

1. Prepare the Toasted Almond Crust (see recipe on p. 118) in a 9-inch springform pan. Follow the recipe as directed.

2. Prepare the Flan batter (see recipe on p. 94). Follow the recipe as directed.

3. Preheat the oven to 280°F. Generously grease and flour the springform pan (see Trade Secret on p. 76). Fill the springform pan with the Flan batter and place it on a baking sheet.

4. Place the baking sheet in the center of the oven, directly on the middle shelf. Bake for 35 to 40 minutes, until the cake is slightly firm to the touch and jiggles in the center (this is a shallow cake, so it shouldn't soufflé much). If at the end of this baking time, the cake is starting to soufflé but still has a loose center, reduce the oven temperature to 250°F and bake for another 8 to 10 minutes. Remove from the oven and set aside to cool to room temperature, about 1 hour.

5. Refrigerate for 1 hour to cool the cake completely.

6. Loosen the cheesecake from the springform pan by sliding an offset spatula around the inside ring. Remove the springform pan from the cake and transfer to a plate. Refrigerate for at least 8 hours or overnight before decorating.

7. Prepare the Salted Caramel (see recipe on p. 128). Set aside while still warm, but not hot.

8. Pour the Salted Caramel on the center of the cake. Using the back of a wooden spoon or a silicone offset spatula, spread the caramel evenly over the top of the cake, being careful not to spread over the cake's edge.

9. While the caramel is still warm, press the toasted almonds into it. Work quickly! As caramel cools, it becomes less sticky and decorations do not adhere as well. Sprinkle with the sea salt crystals.

10. Transfer to the freezer for 2 to 3 hours before slicing.

11. Slice the cake with a thin, nonserrated knife that is dipped in hot water and wiped dry after each slice. Serve immediately or store in the freezer well wrapped for up to 3 months.

ELI'S TRADE SECRET *Toasting the almonds in this recipe at a low temperature for a long time produces a deeper, richer flavor.*

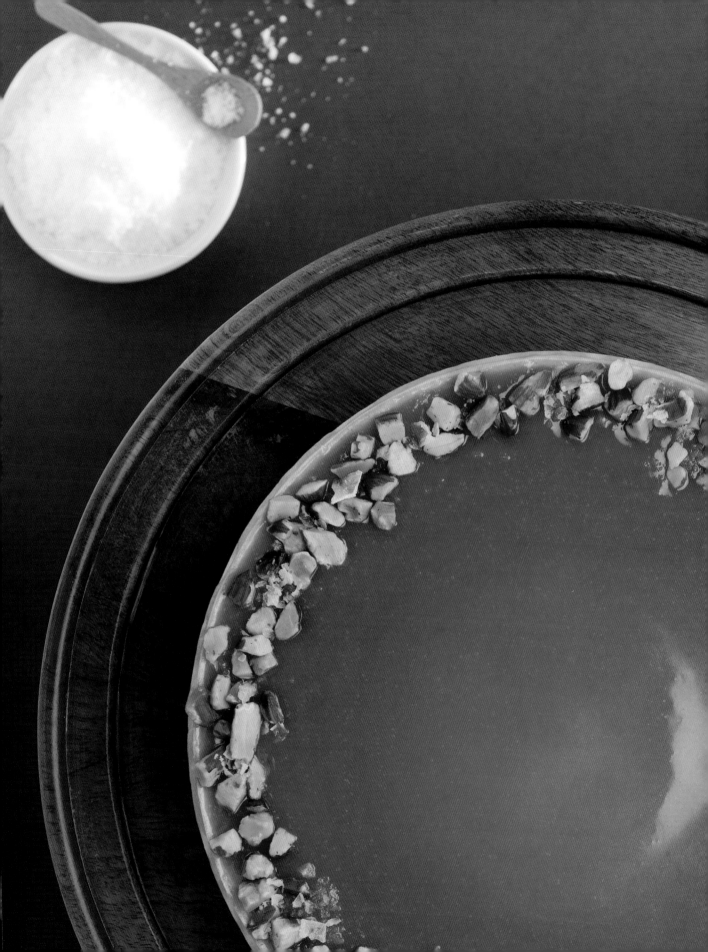

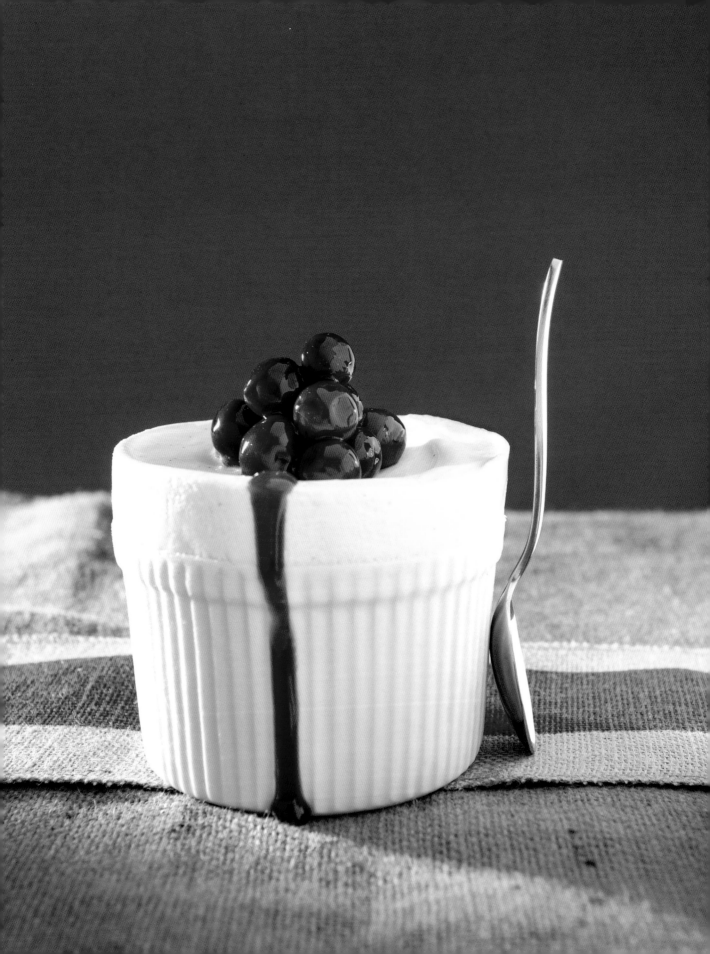

Vanilla Soufflé Glacé with Cherry Compote

YIELD: 2 (8-INCH) ROUND DEEP RAMEKINS

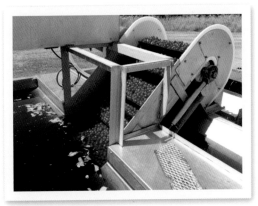

Just-picked Montmorency cherries at Sill Farms.
PHOTO BY JEFF ANDERSON

Third-generation family-owned Sill Farms, in the heart of southwestern Michigan's lush fruit belt, supplies our Montmorency cherries. Our cherries are picked at the peak of ripeness and offer the perfect sweet–tart flavor to complement the rich, creamy mascarpone cheese. This is an unbaked dessert. We recommend using a thermometer when making the sabayon to ensure that the egg yolks are heated to a safe temperature of 150°F.

Shopping List

FOR THE VANILLA SOUFFLÉ GLACÉ:

10 large egg yolks, room temperature

3 large egg whites

1 cup granulated sugar, divided

1 (8-ounce) package mascarpone cheese

2 cups heavy whipping cream

2 whole vanilla beans

1 teaspoon vanilla extract

FOR THE CHERRY COMPOTE:

4½ cups (20 ounces) pitted fresh or frozen thawed Bing cherries

1 cup brandy or orange juice

½ cup granulated sugar

1. Prepare the Vanilla Soufflé Glacé (see recipe on p. 107). Follow the recipe as directed.

2. Prepare the Cherry Compote (see recipe on p. 126). Follow the recipe as directed.

3. Serve the Vanilla Soufflé Glacé straight from the freezer with the Cherry Compote spooned over the top of each serving.

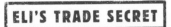

ELI'S TRADE SECRET *To achieve the fluffiest egg whites, make sure your bowl is completely clean and grease free. Try washing it with a capful of vinegar and a sprinkle of salt.*

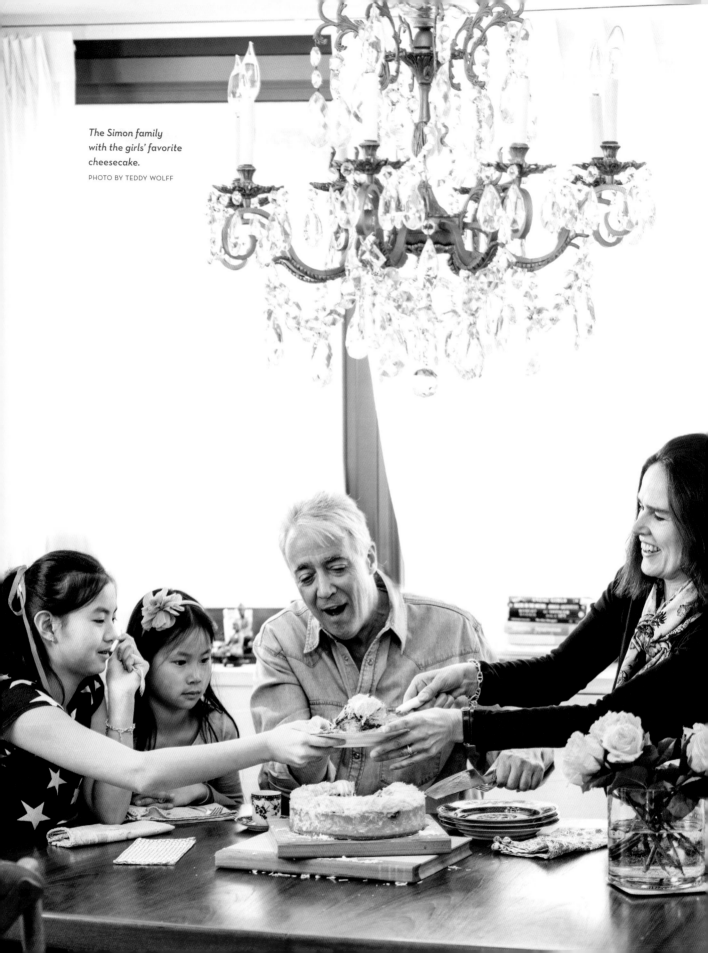

The Simon family with the girls' favorite cheesecake.
PHOTO BY TEDDY WOLFF

White Chocolate Cheesecake with Raspberries and Nutella

YIELD: 1 (9-INCH) SPRINGFORM CHEESECAKE PAN / 12 SERVINGS

In addition to his well-known role as the host of Weekend Edition Saturday *on NPR, Scott Simon is a television personality, an author, and a big Eli's cheesecake fan, and he and his wife, Caroline, have plenty of warm memories that feature our delicious desserts. Recently, their oldest daughter, Elise, found out that she needed braces. Since many of her friends had them as well, she was excited about it—until she heard that she wouldn't be allowed to eat popcorn and caramel once she got them.*

"Wait!" she said. "You mean no *Salted Caramel Cheesecake??" Elise was willing to put up with tightening wires and snapping bands—but no Salted Caramel Cheesecake? Forget it.*

Through dutiful trial and error, Elise discovered that it's possible to fork a bite of Salted Caramel Cheesecake into the back of her mouth, avoiding the danger zone. ("Just be sure to floss carefully," adds her dad.)

When we asked Elise and her younger sister, Paulina, to come up with their favorite cheesecake, the girls took the job seriously: They conducted a poll of their classmates in the second and sixth grades at their Washington, DC schools. The clear winner: White Chocolate Cheesecake with Raspberries and Nutella.

Shopping List

FOR THE CHOCOLATE CRUMB CRUST:

1½ cups (16 ounces) finely ground chocolate wafer crumbs

¼ cup confectioners' sugar

¼ cup unsalted butter, melted

FOR THE WHITE CHOCOLATE GANACHE:

5 squares (5 ounces) Baker's Premium White Chocolate

½ cup heavy cream

FOR THE WHITE CHOCOLATE AND NUTELLA BATTER:

3½ (8-ounce) packages cream cheese, room temperature

1 cup granulated sugar

3 tablespoons cake flour

½ teaspoon salt

2 large whole eggs, room temperature

2 large egg yolks, room temperature

1 cup melted Nutella or other hazelnut spread

FOR THE GARNISH:

2 cups fresh raspberries, washed and dried

RECIPE CONTINUES ON PAGE 200

WHITE CHOCOLATE CHEESECAKE WITH RASPBERRIES AND NUTELLA *(CONTINUED FROM PAGE 199)*

(CONTINUED FROM PAGE 199)

1. Prepare the Chocolate Crumb Crust (see recipe on p. 116) in a 9-inch springform pan. Follow the recipe as directed.

2. Prepare the White Chocolate Ganache (see recipe on p. 103). Follow the recipe as directed.

3. Prepare the White Chocolate and Nutella batter (see recipe variation on p. 102). Follow the recipe as directed.

4. Preheat the oven to 300°F. Generously grease and flour the springform pan (see Trade Secret on p. 76). Fill the springform pan with the White Chocolate and Nutella batter. Using an offset spatula, smooth down the batter until it is level.

5. Place the filled springform pan in the center of the oven, directly on the middle shelf. Bake for 40 to 50 minutes, until the cake is firm to the touch around the edges. Give the cake a gentle shake. The baking time is complete if the center of the cake jiggles. Remove from the oven and set aside to cool to room temperature, about 1 hour.

6. Refrigerate for at least 1 hour before removing the cake from the pan.

7. Loosen the cheesecake from the springform pan by sliding an offset spatula around the inside ring. Remove the springform pan from the cake and transfer to a serving plate. Refrigerate 8 hours or overnight before serving.

8. Before serving, decorate the cake by placing the fresh raspberries on the top of the cake. Transfer to the freezer for 2 to 3 hours before slicing.

9. Slice the cake with a thin, nonserrated knife that is dipped in hot water and wiped dry after each slice. Serve immediately or store in the freezer well wrapped for up to 3 months.

200   *THE ELI'S CHEESECAKE COOKBOOK*

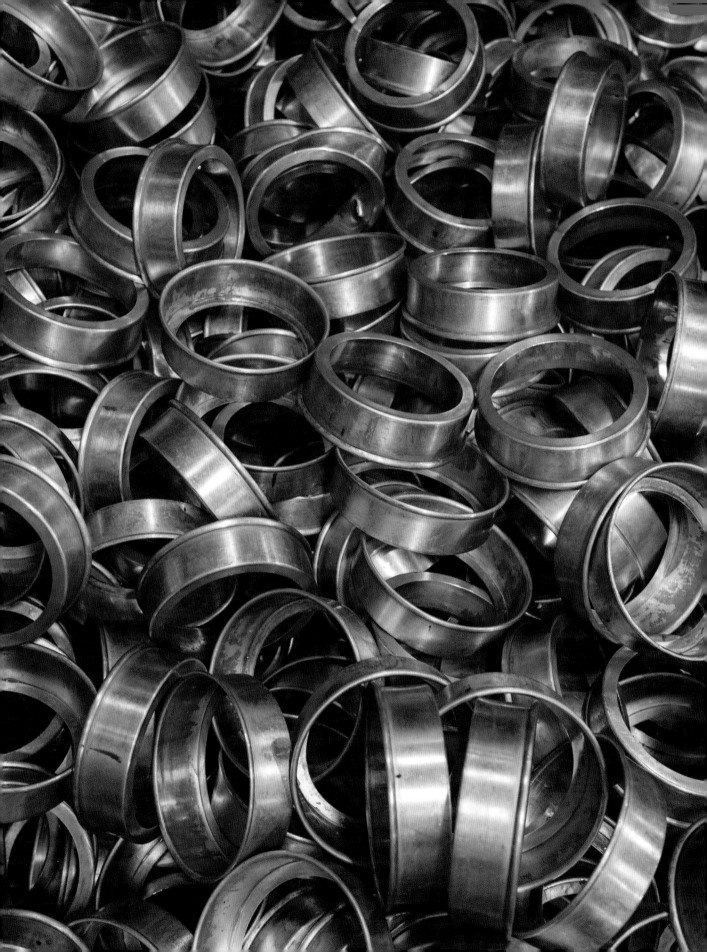

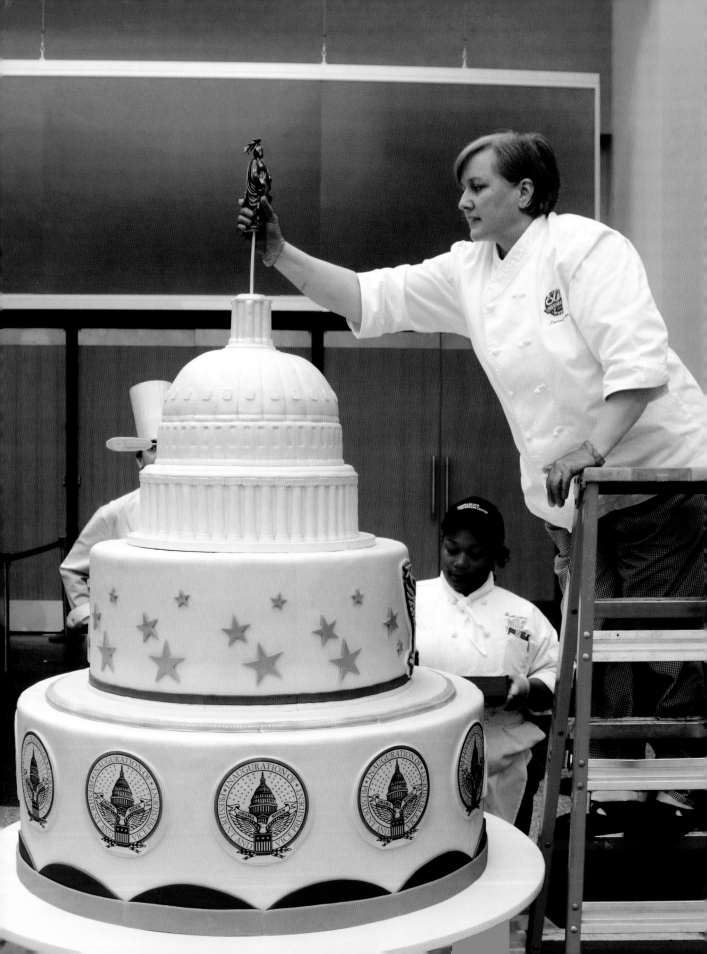

CELEBRATORY CAKES BIG AND SMALL

"IT'S A HELLUVA CAKE!" That's what Eli said as he stepped back and admired the huge cake he'd made for Chicago's 150th birthday celebration. Eli's Cheesecake has been baking up giant celebratory cakes for most of its 35-year history! The Office of the Mayor refers to Eli's cheesecakes as "a symbol of the city" and "an ambassador of Chicago's culinary scene."

"Marc has turned his father's classic old Chicago cheesecake into a civic pillar. Chicago's mayor famously sends Eli's cheesecakes rather than dead fish; Eli's cheesecakes have nourished inauguration balls," wrote Scott Simon in his book *Unforgettable*. No celebration is complete without a big Eli's cheesecake.

Marc recalled about one of his favorite Big Cakes, "It is heartbreakingly rare for a Chicago baseball team to win the World Series. It has been over 108 years for the Chicago Cubs, but the White Sox broke a nearly century-long losing streak in 2005 when they took home the title. Chicagoans went crazy when the White Sox won. Over one million people filled the streets to watch the victory parade. The next day, team owner Jerry Reinsdorf and manager Ozzie Guillen came to City Hall to present the World Series trophy to Mayor Daley and the City Council. But first there was a stop in the lobby of City Hall, where I introduced the Mayor, Ozzie, and Reinsdorf and presented them with a giant World Series victory cheesecake. It doesn't get any better than that! My dad, a lifelong White Sox fan, would have been so proud."

You might wonder what goes into such a big cake. The mind-boggling grocery list for the 2,000-pound cakes Eli's has prepared for President Clinton's and President Obama's inauguration celebrations included 1,330 pounds of cream cheese, 300 pounds of sugar, 150 dozen eggs, 65 pounds of sour cream, 100 pounds of buttercream frosting, and 100 pounds of marzipan.

For *slightly* smaller celebrations—like family birthdays, dinner parties, and dessert buffets—a couple of clever ideas follow that are sure to delight you and your family. The decoration part of these recipes is family friendly, as they've been tested many times by our daughters and their friends since they were only four years old or so. We think making the dessert is as much fun as having the party!

Eli's executive pastry chef Laurel Boger places an edible bronze Statue of Freedom atop a cheesecake Capitol building for President Obama's Inaugural Staff Ball in 2013.

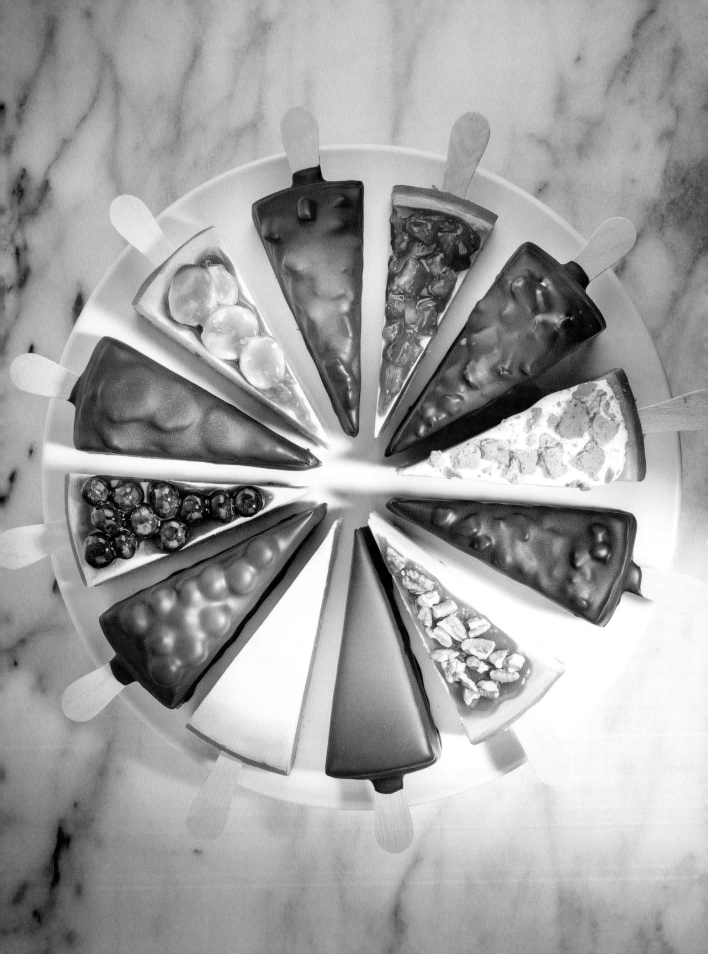

Cheesecake Dippers

YIELD: 1 (9-INCH) SPRINGFORM CHEESECAKE PAN / 12 SERVINGS

Dippers were invented during one really hot Taste of Chicago. We wanted to offer customers a treat that would keep them cool, and we love anything you can eat on a stick. We hand-dip frozen cheesecake slices in chocolate and serve them on a stick for the ultimate forkless dessert.

A fun idea: Throw a dipping party. Your friends can dip slices of cheesecake in chocolate and roll them in their favorite chopped candy or nuts. Everyone gets just what they want!

Shopping List

FOR THE SHORTBREAD CRUST:

1½ sticks (12 tablespoons) cold unsalted butter

½ cup confectioners' sugar

½ teaspoon salt

¼ teaspoon vanilla extract

1½ cups all-purpose flour

FOR THE ORIGINAL PLAIN BATTER:

4 (8-ounce) packages cream cheese, room temperature

1 cup granulated sugar

¼ cup cake flour

2 large whole eggs, room temperature

1 large egg yolk, room temperature

¾ cup sour cream, room temperature

1 teaspoon vanilla extract

¼ teaspoon salt

FOR THE GARNISH:

16 ounces chocolate shell ice cream topping or melted chocolate, kept at 100°F

1 tablespoon vegetable oil

12 wooden sticks

Candy, nuts, or holiday sprinkles, as desired

Check out this photo for ideas for your own Cheesecake Dippers (see recipe on the following page).

RECIPE CONTINUES ON PAGE 206

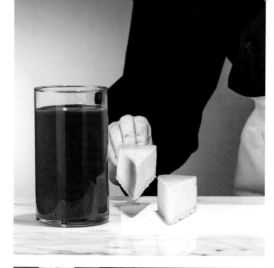

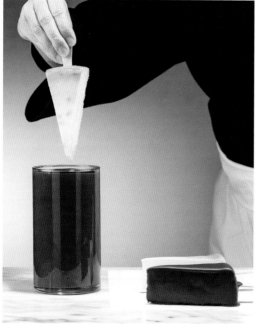

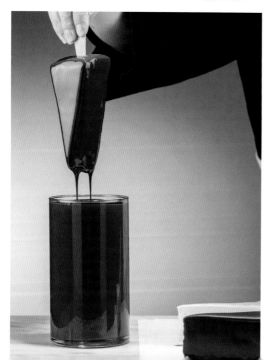

CHEESECAKE DIPPERS

(CONTINUED FROM PAGE 205)

1. Prepare the Shortbread Crust (see recipe on p. 110) in a 9-inch springform pan. Follow the recipe as directed.

2. Prepare the Original Plain batter (see recipe on p. 78). Follow the recipe as directed.

3. Preheat the oven to 375°F. Generously grease and flour the springform pan (see Trade Secret on p. 76). Fill the springform pan with the Original Plain batter.

4. Place the filled springform pan in the center of the oven, directly on the middle shelf. Bake for 15 minutes, then rotate the cake 180 degrees to ensure even browning. (All ovens bake differently, so be alert for hot spots in your own oven.)

5. Bake for 15 minutes more, and again rotate the cake 180 degrees. The cake should be starting to soufflé and should be light in color. Continue to bake for 10 minutes more, for a total of 40 minutes at 375°F.

6. Reduce the oven temperature to 250°F. The cake should be golden brown and lightly souffléd on the sides. Leave the cake in the oven for 10 minutes more. (This step and the two that follow allow the cake to cool to room temperature gently, preventing cracking.) Give the cake a gentle shake; it is done if the center of the cake jiggles and the surface of the cake is slightly firm. Turn the oven off and open the oven door wide. Leave the cake in the oven for 10 minutes more. Remove from the oven and set aside to cool to room temperature, about 1 hour.

7. Loosen the cheesecake from the springform pan by sliding an offset spatula around the inside ring. Remove the springform pan from the cake and transfer to a plate. Refrigerate for at least 8 hours or overnight before serving.

8. Slice the cake into 12 slices with a thin, nonserrated knife that is dipped in hot water and wiped dry after each slice. Transfer to the freezer for 30 minutes.

9. Remove from the freezer and insert 1 4-inch wooden stick halfway into the heel of each slice. Return to the freezer for 2 to 3 hours, until the sticks are frozen and secure in each slice.

10. Place the chocolate shell ice cream topping or melted chocolate in a tall, cylindrical container. Remove the cake from the freezer and place it next to a large sheet of parchment paper. Dip each cake slice directly into the chocolate and then transfer it to the parchment paper, sliding the slice out of the puddle a bit to remove any excess chocolate.

11. Before the chocolate on each Dipper sets, invert it and sprinkle with your choice of candy, nuts, or holiday sprinkles. Serve immediately or store in the freezer well wrapped for up to 3 months.

VARIATION

Banana Cheesecake Dippers: This is just the ultimate! Follow the recipe as directed but use the Banana batter instead of the Original Plain. This recipe tastes as good as it looks. Have fun enrobing!

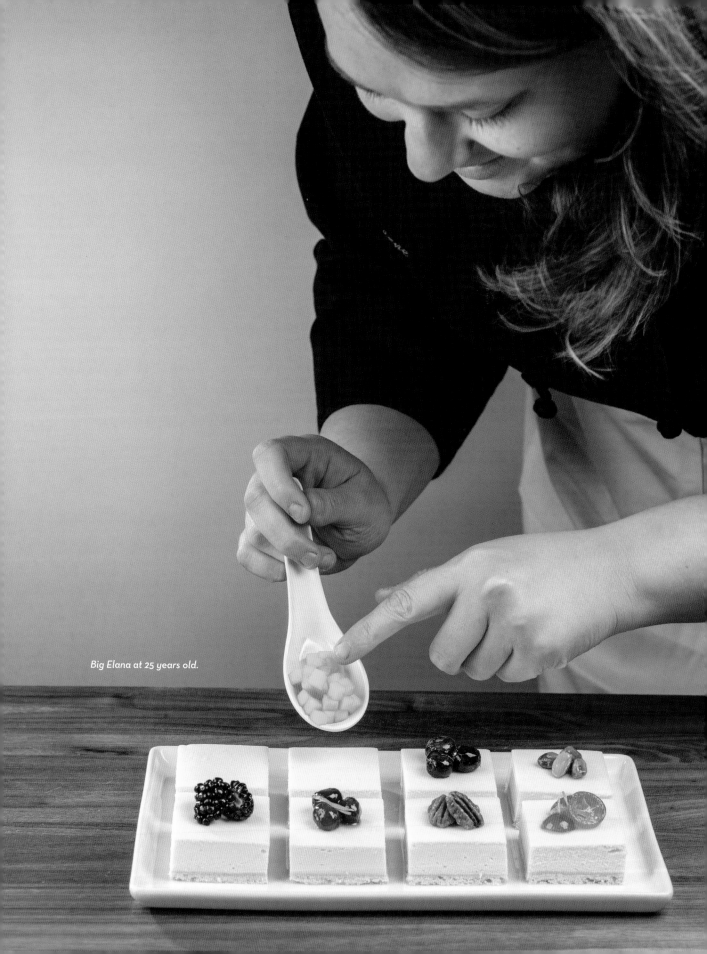

Big Elana at 25 years old.

Original Plain Cuties

YIELD: 24 (2-INCH) SQUARE CUTIES

One day when our daughter Elana was nine years old, she was sitting in the back seat of the our big red minivan and suddenly announced, "Let's make little cheesecakes and call them Cuties. You know, like a box of candy...only cheesecake." That really happened...it's on video.

Cuties turned out to be a really versatile size. They're perfect for dessert buffets or hostess gifts, enrobed in chocolate, as an amuse bouche...or even splashed with espresso! They're so small, they're practically guilt free.

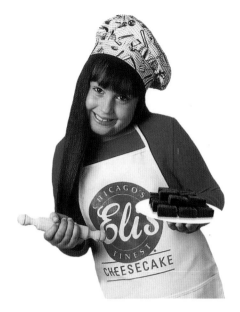

Little Elana at 9 years old.

Shopping List

FOR THE SHORTBREAD CRUST:

1½ sticks (12 tablespoons) cold unsalted butter

½ cup confectioners' sugar

½ teaspoon salt

¼ teaspoon vanilla extract

1½ cups all-purpose flour

FOR THE ORIGINAL PLAIN BATTER:

4 (8-ounce) packages cream cheese, room temperature

1 cup granulated sugar

¼ cup cake flour

2 large whole eggs, room temperature

1 large egg yolk, room temperature

¾ cup sour cream, room temperature

1 teaspoon vanilla extract

¼ teaspoon salt

RECIPE CONTINUES ON PAGE 211

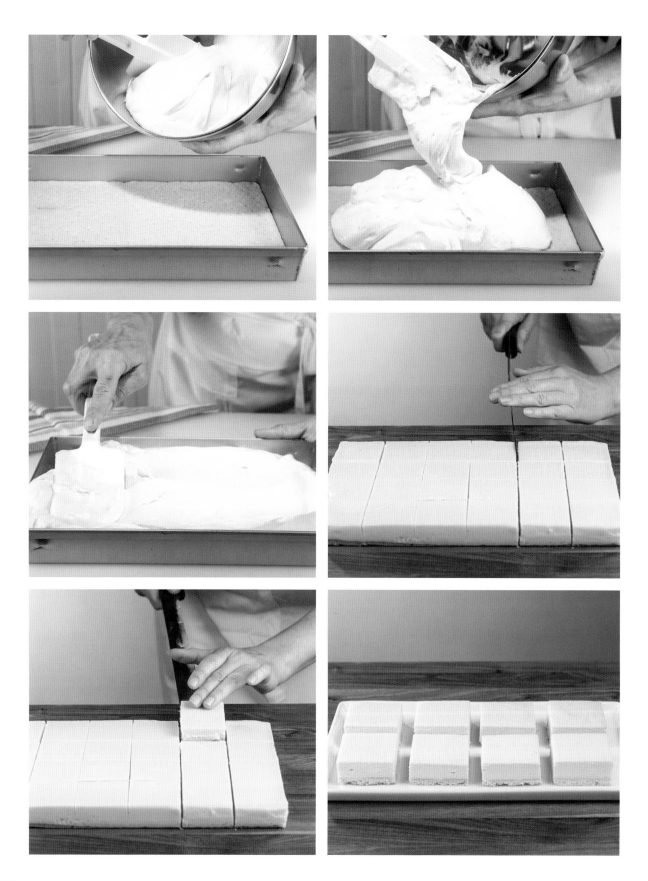

ORIGINAL PLAIN CUTIES

(CONTINUED FROM PAGE 209)

1. Prepare the Shortbread Crust (see recipe on p. 110) in a 9- × 13-inch pan. Follow the recipe as directed.

2. Prepare the Original Plain batter (see recipe on p. 78). Follow the recipe as directed.

3. Preheat the oven to 275°F. Generously grease and flour the springform pan (see Trade Secret on p. 76). Fill the 9- × 13-inch pan with the Original Plain batter.

4. Place the filled pan in the center of the oven, directly on the middle shelf. Bake for 30 to 35 minutes, until firm to the touch in the center. The cake should appear colorless and should remain level. Remove from the oven and set aside to cool to room temperature, about 1 hour.

5. Loosen the cheesecake from the pan by sliding an offset spatula around the outside rim of the pan. Refrigerate for at least 8 hours or overnight.

6. Transfer to the freezer for 2 to 3 hours before slicing.

7. Slice the cake into 2-inch cubes with a thin, nonserrated knife that is dipped in hot water and wiped dry after each slice. Serve immediately or store in the freezer well wrapped for up to 3 months.

VARIATIONS ON PAGE 212

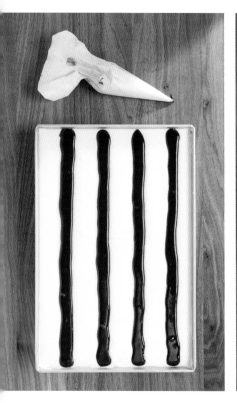
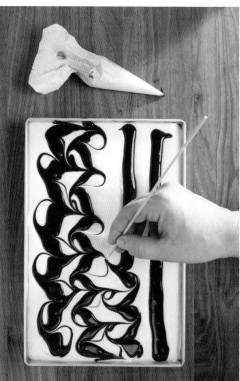
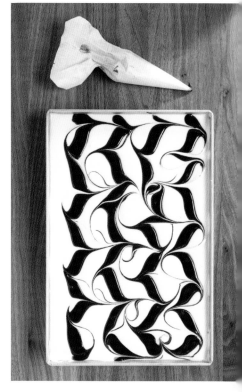

ORIGINAL PLAIN CUTIES

(CONTINUED FROM PAGE 211)

VARIATIONS

Swirl Ganache Cheesecake Cuties: Before baking the Original Plain batter, pipe four horizontal lines of Belgian Chocolate Ganache (see recipe on p. 83) onto the surface of the batter. Using the handle of a spoon, swirl the piped Ganache into a decorative "S" pattern.

Cheesecake Cutie Sandwich: Gather all your cookie cutters. Start with your favorite cookie recipes or try baking our Chocolate Shortbread Crust (see recipe on p. 113) cut out in your favorite shapes. Warm the cookie cutters before cutting matching shapes from the frozen cheesecake.

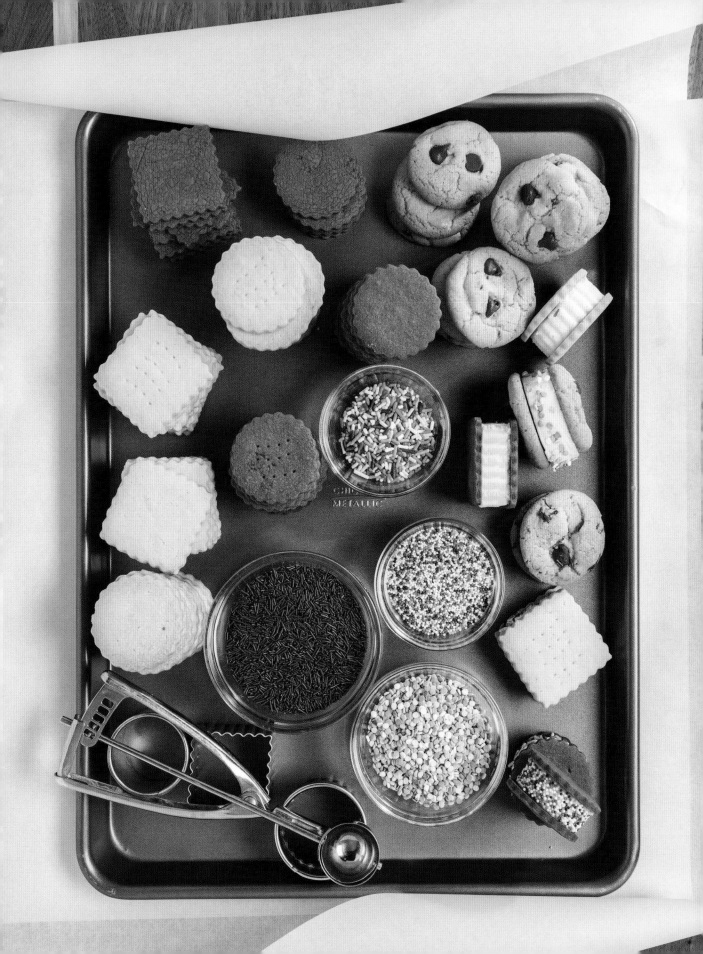

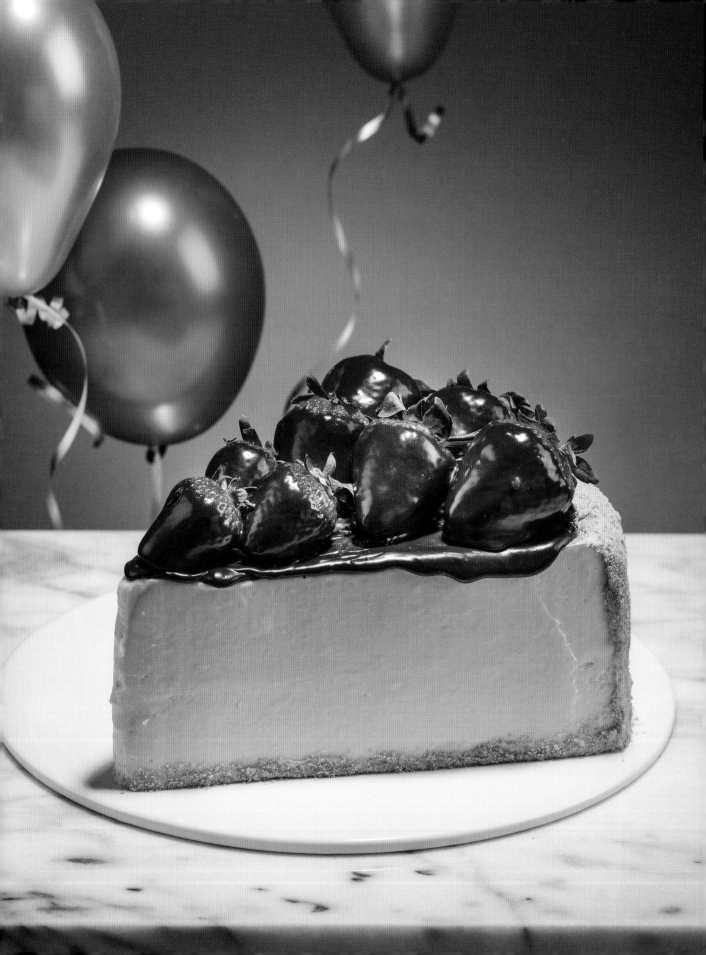

Big-Slice Birthday Cake

YIELD: 1 DOUBLE-HEIGHT (9-INCH) CHEESECAKE /
15 TO 20 SERVINGS

The first time we made a Big-Slice cake was in the 1990s, when Mayor Daley wagered an Eli's Cheesecake during one of the Chicago Bulls' early championships. We've been making them ever since.

This is a great party idea—we make one every year for our daughter Haley's birthday. Invite 20 of your best friends over and have a dessert party. It makes a great photo op!

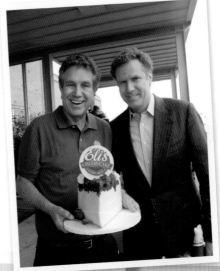

Shopping List

FOR THE SHORTBREAD CRUSTS:

1½ sticks (12 tablespoons) cold unsalted butter

½ cup confectioners' sugar

½ teaspoon salt

¼ teaspoon vanilla extract

1½ cups all-purpose flour

FOR THE ORIGINAL PLAIN BATTER (2 RECIPES REQUIRED):

8 (8-ounce) packages cream cheese, room temperature

2 cups granulated sugar

½ cup cake flour

½ teaspoon salt

4 large whole eggs, room temperature

2 large egg yolks, room temperature

1½ cups sour cream, room temperature

2 teaspoons vanilla extract

FOR THE FROSTING AND GARNISHES:

1 pint fresh whole strawberries

1 cup melted chocolate, for dipping strawberries

3 cups of your favorite frosting

1 cup (16 ounces) graham cracker crumbs

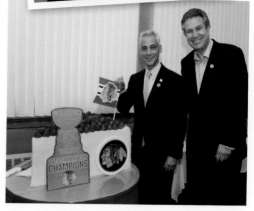

FROM TOP: *Marc stands with his lookalike, Will Ferrell, alongside a Big-Slice cake prepared for Ferrell's Chicago visit to promote his movie The Campaign.*

Chicago's Big Cheese, Mayor Rahm Emanuel, and Marc celebrate the Blackhawks' 2015 victory with the giant slice.

RECIPE CONTINUES ON PAGE 216

BIG-SLICE BIRTHDAY CAKE

(CONTINUED FROM PAGE 215)

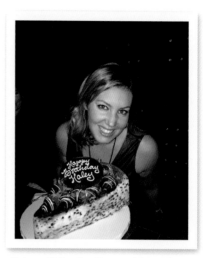

Haley with her Big-Slice Birthday Cake.

1. Prepare the Shortbread Crusts (see recipe on p. 110) in two 9-inch springform pans. Follow the recipe as directed.

2. Prepare enough Original Plain batter to make 2 cakes (see recipe on p. 78). Follow the recipe as directed.

3. Preheat the oven to 375°F. Generously grease and flour the springform pan (see Trade Secret on p. 76). Fill the prepared springform pans with the Original Plain batter. Using an offset spatula, smooth down the batter until it is level.

4. Place the filled springform pans in the center of the oven, directly on the middle shelf. Bake for 15 minutes, then rotate the cakes 180 degrees to ensure even browning. (All ovens bake differently, so be alert for hot spots in your own oven.) The cakes should be starting to soufflé and should be light in color. Continue to bake for 10 minutes more, for a total of 40 minutes at 375°F.

5. Reduce the oven temperature to 250°F and leave the oven door slightly ajar. The cakes should be golden brown and lightly souffléd on the sides. Leave the cakes in the oven for 10 minutes more. (This step and the two that follow allow the cakes to cool to room temperature gently, preventing cracking.) Give the cakes a gentle shake; they are done if the centers of the cakes jiggle and the surfaces of the cakes are slightly firm. Turn the oven off and open the oven door wide. Leave the cakes in the oven for 10 minutes more. Remove from the oven and set aside to cool to room temperature, about 1 hour.

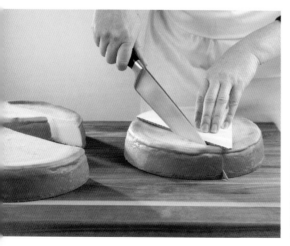
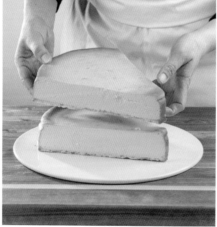
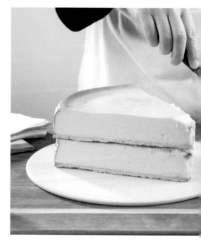

6. Loosen the cheesecakes from the springform pans by sliding an offset spatula around their inside rings. Remove the springform pans from the cakes and transfer to plates. Refrigerate for at least 8 hours or overnight.

7. Wash and dry the strawberries and dip them in the melted chocolate. Set aside on waxed paper to allow the chocolate to harden. Transfer to the freezer for 2 to 3 hours before slicing.

8. Make a paper template of a large triangular slice to set on top of the finished cake. Using a thin, nonserrated knife that is dipped in hot water and wiped dry after each slice, cut the slice shape out of the two cheesecakes' centers.

9. Assemble the two cakes together by stacking them, one on top of the other. Frost the assembled cake using the frosting of your choice. Coat the "crust" of the large slice with the graham cracker crumbs. Garnish with the chocolate-covered strawberries and serve immediately or store in the freezer well wrapped for up to 3 months.

ELI'S TRADE SECRET *Be sure that both cheesecakes are completely frozen before cutting the template slice to make sure it's nice and clean.*

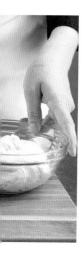
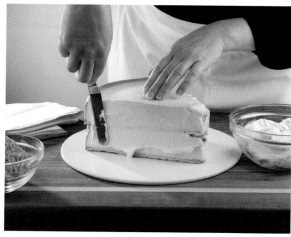
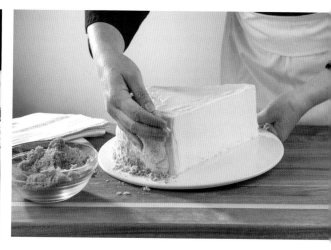

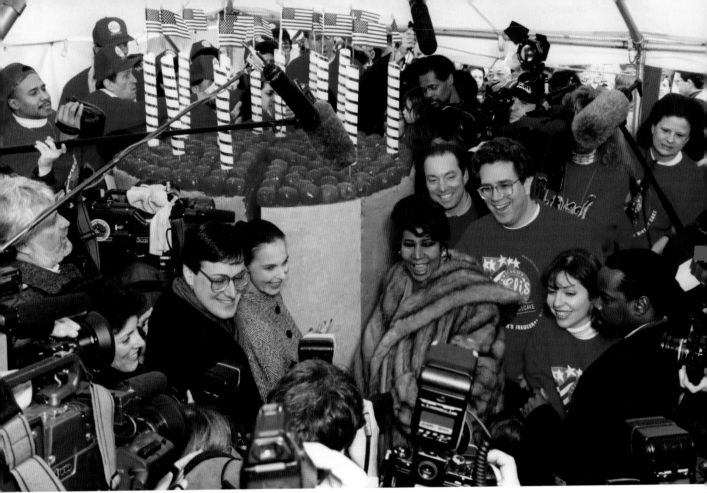

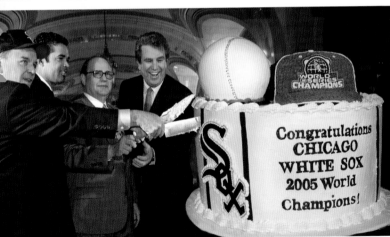

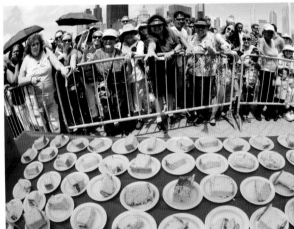

TOP: *Eli's Cheesecake is one of President Clinton's favorite desserts! It was served at the White House and aboard Air Force One. (Of course, now President Clinton is a vegan...but don't worry, Eli's makes vegan cheesecake, so we have him covered.) Eli's made a 2,000-pound cheesecake for both of the Clinton inaugural celebrations in Washington, DC. Pictured here is the Queen of Soul, Aretha Franklin, cutting Clinton's first Inaugural cheesecake at Reunion on the Mall.*

BOTTOM, LEFT: *Left to right: Mayor Richard M. Daley, White Sox manager Ozzie Guillen, White Sox owner Jerry Reinsdorf, and Marc Schulman cut the giant cheesecake created when the White Sox won the World Series in 2005.*

BOTTOM, RIGHT: *Eli's fans line up for a piece of the big cake.*

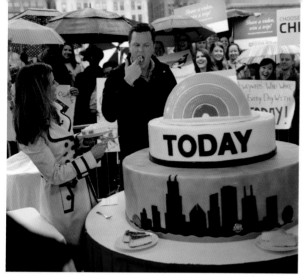

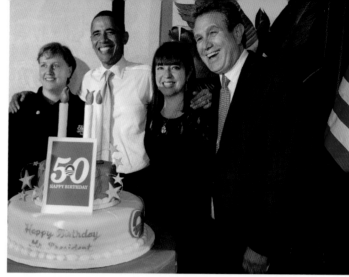

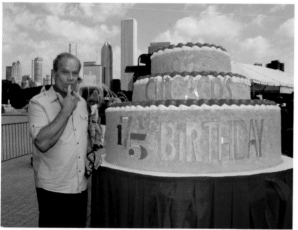

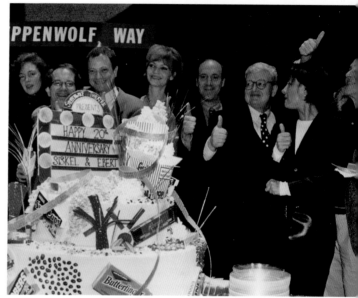

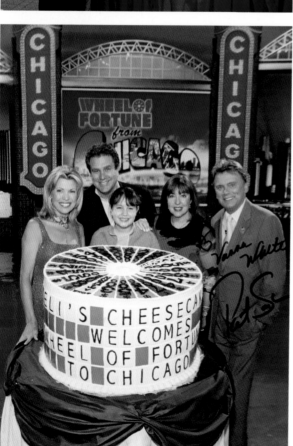

CLOCKWISE FROM TOP LEFT

In 2014, Eli's Cheesecake welcomed the Today Show to Chicago! Shown are hosts Natalie Morales and Willie Geist.

President Obama with his 50th birthday cheesecake. Left to right, Laurel Boger and Maureen and Marc Schulman.

This movie-themed cheesecake was designed for Siskel and Ebert's 20th anniversary, held at the Steppenwolf Theater. Cutting the cake are Martha Lavey, Alan Wilder, Gary Sinise, Joan Allen, Gene Siskel, Roger Ebert, Laurie Metcalf, and John Mahoney.

Eli's created a giant Wheel of Fortune cake for Vanna White and Pat Sajak when the game show filmed on location in Chicago. Also pictured: Maureen, Marc, and Elana Schulman.

Kelsey Grammer, "Mayor of Chicago" on the Starz series Boss, cut the 1,500-pound cheesecake celebrating Chicago's 175th birthday.

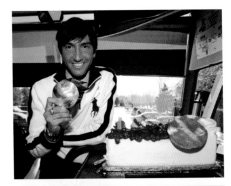

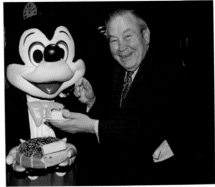

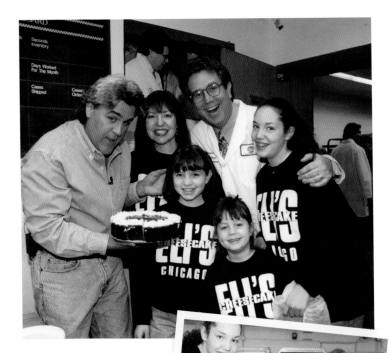

FROM TOP: *Olympic gold medalist and Dancing with the Stars alum Evan Lysacek poses with a Big-Slice cake created to celebrate Evan Lysacek Day in his hometown of Naperville, Illinois.*

Every mouse likes cheese, but Mickey (shown with Eli) got an upgrade: cheesecake.

During a 1996 broadcast of Jay Leno's Tonight Show from Chicago, an actor portraying Marc took Jay into Eli's bakery and told him they'd put his face on every cheesecake made that day—and proceeded to push his face into the entire production line of cakes.

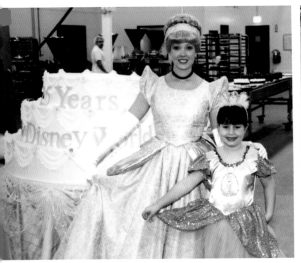

Cinderella and her sidekick, Elana, visit Eli's Bakery before the Cinderella Cheesecake was presented for Disney World's 25th Anniversary.

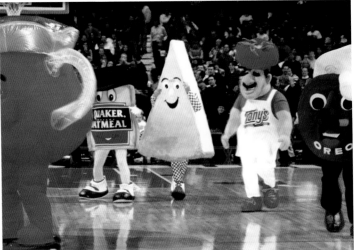

The Slice, Eli's Cheesecake's mascot, was center court at the United Center; Marc was inside the suit!

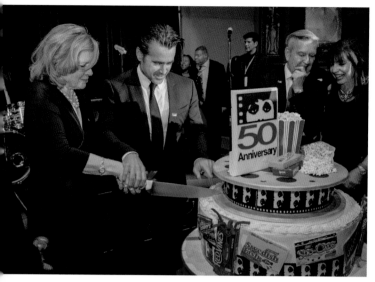

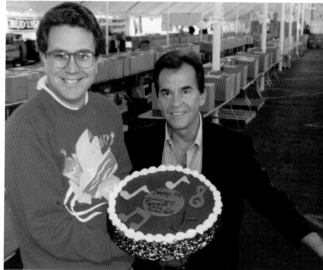

ABOVE LEFT: *For the Chicago International Film Festival's 50th anniversary, Colin Farrell and Liv Ullmann were on hand to cut our massive movie-themed cheesecake, complete with popcorn, favorite movie candies, and a white chocolate film reel. Also pictured are Michael Kutza, founder of the Chicago International Film Festival, and Maureen Schulman.*

ABOVE RIGHT: *Marc Schulman and Dick Clark at the Les Turner Foundation ALS Mammoth Music Mart.*

RIGHT: *Emilio and Gloria Estefan and Josh Segarra and Ana Villafane, the actors who portray them in the Broadway-bound show "On Your Feet," get ready to dive into a giant Eli's Tres Leches cake at the show's Broadway in Chicago opening night party.*

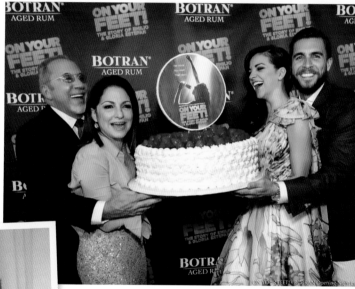

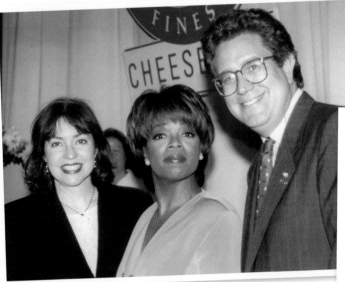

Slice of Heaven

"Maybe it's the all-butter cookie crust, maybe it's the Madagascar bourbon vanilla beans—this cheesecake is perfection on a plate."
($28, Eli's Cheesecake; elicheesecake.com)

At a Harpo Studios event, Maureen and Marc served Eli's Cheesecake, and Oprah Winfrey stopped by. Later, she called Eli's Original Plain "perfection on a plate" in the pages of O, The Oprah Magazine.

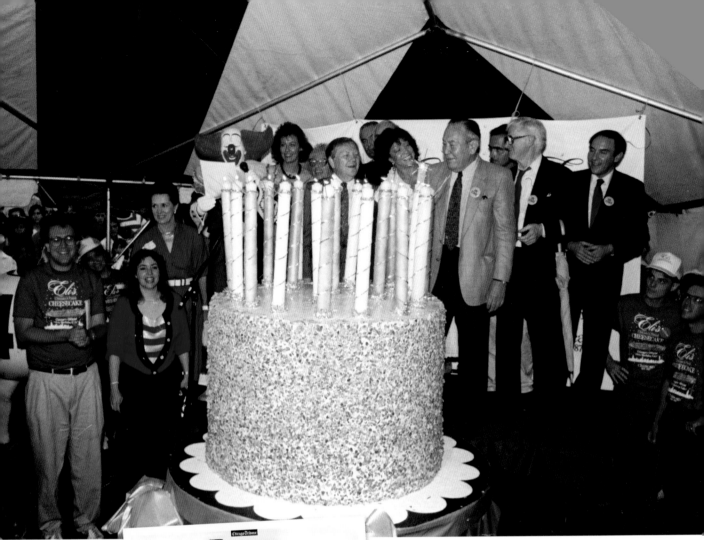

Eli lighting the candles on his first Big Cheesecake, made to celebrate Chicago's 150th birthday in 1987.

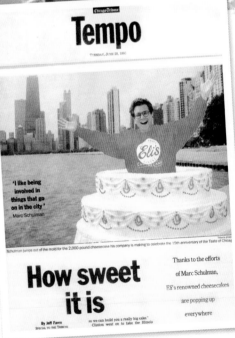

Marc pops out of a giant cake in this Chicago Tribune feature.

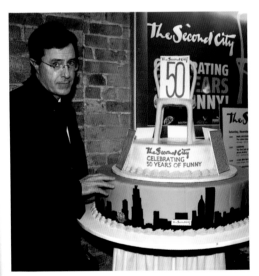

Second City alum Stephen Colbert deadpans next to Eli's 50 Years of Funny cheesecake.

Eli frosts the first big cheesecake ever, which weighed in at 1,000 pounds and was served free to the public at Taste of Chicago.

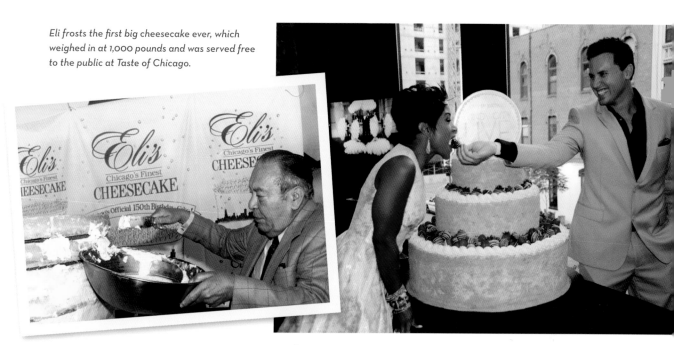

Windy City Live's Ryan Chiaverini gives co-host Val Warner a taste of an Eli's Cheesecake made to celebrate the show's first anniversary.

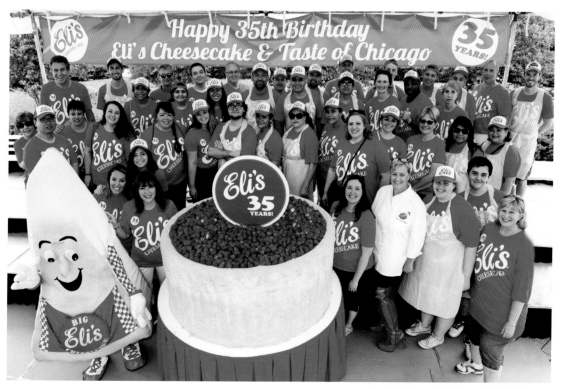

The Eli's team celebrating the 35th birthday at Taste of Chicago with a 1,500-pound cheesecake, which was served free to the public. Laurel Boger (first row, third from right) wears glam boots in honor of the event's guest stars, the cast of the musical Kinky Boots.

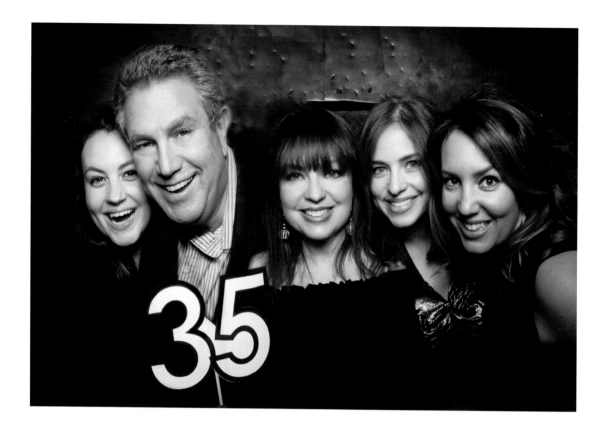

From our family to yours:

We hope you have fun making all of our favorite recipes from Eli's The Place For Steak
and The Eli's Cheesecake Bakery. Thanks for being an Eli's fan!

Thank you!

Antonio Rivera; Armando Chavez; Aurelio Ayala; Fidel Becerril; Fidel Mar Espino; Haley, Kori, and
Elana Schulman; Juanita Chajon; Judith Ghalioungui; Lisa Ripka; Marc Schulman; Maria Santonato;
Marina and Jorge Cotaquispe; Mary Gale; Rod Hunter; and Scott Brewer. The Eli's team would like to
give an especially big thank you to Sarah Duff Zupancic and Laurel Boger for all their hard work!

PHOTOS: Jeff Anderson, Jennifer Girard, Kingen Smith, K Shack, Leigh Loftus, Maureen Schulman,
Michelle Reed, Peter McCullough, Petr Bednarik, Richard Shay, Robert E. Potter III, Steve Leonard,
Steve Somen, Teddy Wolff, Tim Klein, and Vito Palmisano.

INDEX

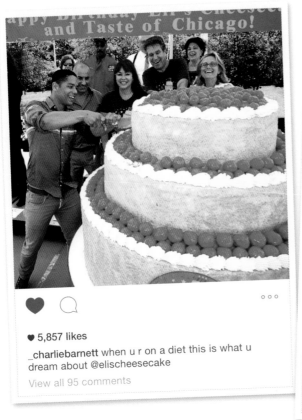

❤ 🗨   ○○○

❤ **5,857 likes**

_charliebarnett when u r on a diet this is what u
dream about @elischeesecake

View all 95 comments

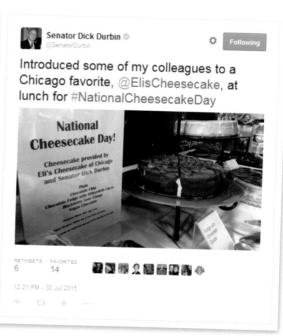

Senator Dick Durbin ✔
@SenatorDurbin

⚙   Following

Introduced some of my colleagues to a
Chicago favorite, @ElisCheesecake, at
lunch for #NationalCheesecakeDay

RETWEETS   FAVORITES
6   14

12:21 PM - 30 Jul 2015

ABOUT THE AUTHORS

Jolene Worthington, executive vice president of The Eli's Cheesecake Company, is one of America's premier cake and cheesecake bakers. Jolene trained in pastries, baking, and candymaking at the Culinary Institute of America in Hyde Park, NY. She has lectured on her technique for creating premium cheesecake at the American Institute of Baking and has spoken to the Culinary Historians of Chicago on the "History of Cheesecake." Before joining Eli's, Jolene wrote the "Cooks' Tools" column for the *Chicago Tribune*, was the culinary consultant for the Time–Life cookbook series *Good Cooks,* and was a freelance writer for *Cuisine Magazine.* Jolene is a member of the board of directors of Slow Food Chicago, has served on the governing board for the Cooking and Hospitality Institute of Chicago, is a board member of and mentor for the Chicago High School for Agricultural Sciences, and is a member of Les Dames d'Escoffier. Jolene's long-standing passion for food and creative approach to all endeavors make hers a unique voice in the food world.

Diana Moles, vice president of research and development for The Eli's Cheesecake Company, wears two toques—one creative and the other technical. Diana oversees research and development of new products for domestic and foreign markets and directs the process and application of baking technology. Her deep understanding of food science allows her to magically turn concept into reality. Her professional training includes time at the American Institute of Baking and the Culinary Institute of America. An award-winning pastry chef, Diana is also a member of Les Dames d'Escoffier. She teaches cooking and fine pastry classes in the Chicago area and is also an advocate for people with disabilities.

Maureen Schulman, director of publicity for The Eli's Cheesecake Company, is an award-winning publicist and photographer. Maureen has been a part of the Eli's Cheesecake story since 1980, when she joined her father-in-law, Eli Schulman, and husband, Marc, in launching Eli's Cheesecake at its public debut at the first Taste of Chicago. Maureen has given

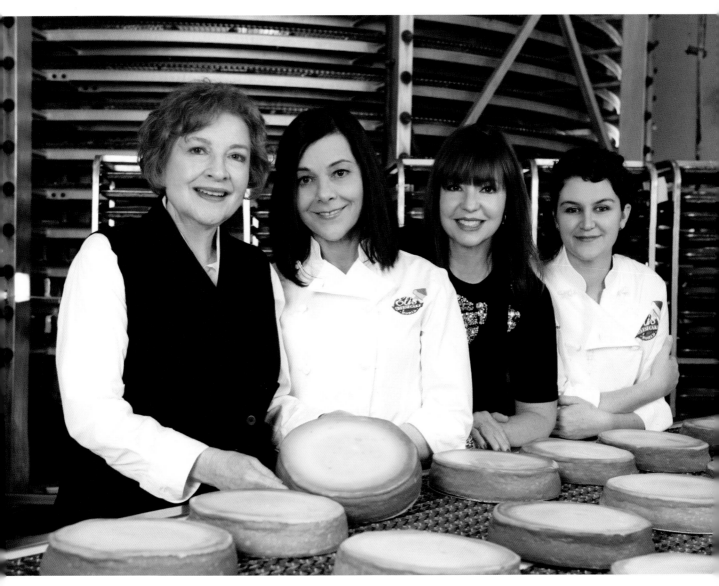

LEFT TO RIGHT: *Jolene Worthington, Diana Moles, Maureen Schulman, and Tara Lane*

significantly of her time to assist not-for-profit organizations: she serves as president of the board of The Happiness Club, a diverse group of Chicago kids who encourage positive values and social change through original hip-hop and pop music and dance, and also sits on the board of the Magnificent Mile Foundation. Maureen is also a presidential appointee to the board of the US Holocaust Memorial Museum. She is a graduate of the University of Miami and received a master's degree in journalism from the Medill School of Northwestern University.

ABOUT THE AUTHORS (CONTINUED)

Tara Lane is an award-winning chef and culinary innovation consultant. Tara apprenticed at New York's renowned François Payard before receiving national acclaim as executive pastry chef at Chicago's Blackbird and Avec restaurants. In addition to undergraduate degrees from Portland's Le Cordon Bleu and the School of the Art Institute in Chicago, Tara earned a M.S. in design methods from the Illinois Institute of Technology. She also served as the food preservationist at the Jane Addams Hull House Kitchen in Chicago, where she focused on food advocacy and policy issues. Tara, a member of Les Dames d'Escoffier, remains committed to seasonality, sustainability, and regionalism.

Peter McCullough is the CEO of McCullough Photo, a photography firm specializing in food, architecture, commercial design, and concept photography. Peter hails from Belfast, Northern Ireland, where he began his career as chef at the award-winning McMasters. He also served as executive sous chef at the Kensington Hilton in London and at the Chicago Hilton and Towers.

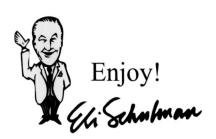

Enjoy!

Eli Schulman